MW00583855

My Dialysis Journey

Gina Novak

ISBN 978-1-63874-466-5 (paperback)
ISBN 978-1-63874-467-2 (digital)

Copyright © 2021 by Gina Novak

All rights reserved. No part of this publication may be reproduced, distributed, or transmitted in any form or by any means, including photocopying, recording, or other electronic or mechanical methods without the prior written permission of the publisher. For permission requests, solicit the publisher via the address below.

Christian Faith Publishing, Inc.
832 Park Avenue
Meadville, PA 16335
www.christianfaithpublishing.com

Bibles Referenced: New International Version (NIV); The Message: The Bible in Contemporary English (MSG); Good News Translation (GNT); English Standard Version (ESV); Amplified Bible (AMP); and King James Version (KJV).

Printed in the United States of America

Foreword

I have been a nurse for over thirty-eight years and have worked as a nurse practitioner in dialysis for nearly twenty years. My role has given me the privilege to share in the trials and triumphs of those diagnosed with chronic kidney disease (CKD). I have learned so much from the patients and families under my care. They inspire me every day with their demonstration of perseverance and resilience while facing the adversities of a chronic illness.

The purpose of this book is

- to share insights on the daily challenges of CKD,
- to serve as a companion for those living with dialysis, and
- to walk this journey in the presence of God.

It is my hope that this book will not only provide education about kidney disease, but more importantly that it would bring a spirit of healing into the many lives affected by CKD.

It is not possible nor my intention to give step-by-step instructions on how to live with chronic kidney disease (CKD). As you read, some weeks described will be far behind and some far ahead of your current situation. The journey is unique to you. However, often in life, we find ourselves linked to others in the most mysterious and unpredictable ways. In these times, it is so very reassuring to know that others have walked similar paths. We can learn through their stories if we stop and listen.

The challenges before you are nearly impossible without hope and love. Fortunately, our Creator, God in heaven, never leaves us alone. You may not know or believe in God, and that is okay. I encourage you to read along anyway, choosing what is helpful for you today. This book was written especially for you. It is to form a bond to the others who have taken the same steps you are now forced to take. It is my hope that in sharing their experience, you will be better equipped, and that you will find comfort in any lingering fear.

For those who know God personally, this is a reminder of how deep and how wide and how far his love reaches, even on this rough terrain that you now find yourself. May you feel his warm embrace as you allow his love to pour out onto you and through you onto others in the most wondrous ways.

Most books related to health practices come with cautionary advisement to check with your physician. This book too highly recommends that you have conversations with your provider about any specific questions. I have done my best to provide you with accurate and up-to-date information, but all care does need to be individualized. I encourage you to discuss your readings with your dialysis care team.

There is a bounty of information on CKD available on the internet. I encourage you to use the resources available to you. I have included a few well-known resources that provide additional information on a variety of topics:

- www.kidney.org/patients/resources
- www.davita.com/dialysis
- www.freseniuskidneycare.com
- www.renalcare.org
- www.niddk.nih.gov/health-information/communication-programs/nkdep
- www.cdc.gov/kidneydisease
- www.annanurse.org/patient-education-resources

Preface

This book has a five-part format.

Each week begins with a personal "snippet" of the experience of dialysis. You will find this italicized and in quotes. Although not the exact words, these scenarios are a compilation of real conversations. These shared thoughts may be helpful and relatable as you experience dialysis.

The next section is weekly expectations that are common among hemodialysis patients. Not everyone follows the same course. My hope is that you will find informative and educational content in each of the outlined weeks.

The question section is to encourage you to process this journey. Naming your concerns, jotting down your ideas, or journaling your inner thoughts can be a healthy tool for expression during this life change.

The information section is to increase your understanding of dialysis, small educational bullets of information that may provide insights or provoke other questions for you to take to your individual care teams.

The scriptures and prayers are to help you lay your burdens at the foot of the cross and feel enveloped in his arms. May God be your safe place in this journey.

Lord, I lift this reader to you right now. I pray that you will meet them in this exact moment and remove this yoke from their necks. I pray for your peace to surround them through every struggle and every celebration. I lift their families, their health care teams, and the ongoing research to improve the treatments for CKD. Thank you for walking toward us, with us, and bringing others alongside of us. Amen.

When I am afraid, I will put my trust in You. (Psalm 56:3)

Chapter 1

In the Beginning

Today I was told that I need to start dialysis. I was told that my diabetes and high blood pressure had caused damage to my kidneys a few years ago.

Hearing this news, my first thought was, "There must be some mistake."

I still make urine a lot. My doctor must be wrong, or there is an error with my blood work. I mean, I really don't feel that bad. A little tired maybe, and I have been nauseated for quite a while, but really that could be just about anything...right?

Even if I do need dialysis, I am sure my kidneys are going to get better. The kidney specialist or nephrologist suggests that I have more blood work immediately.

And then...my nephrologist called to tell me that my blood work results show a worsening in my kidney function. He asked how I was feeling. I'm pretty swollen and short of breath when I walk up the stairs. He wants me to go to the hospital and get a temporary catheter in my chest so that I can start dialysis this week.

Well, at least it's just a temporary catheter, which sounds like my kidneys will get better.

Truthfully, I'm scared.

Week 1

You have just been handed some devastating news. Your kidneys are failing, and soon you will need dialysis! What does that even mean?

Common thoughts that may occur in these moments are:

- *But I still make urine. Why do I need dialysis?*
- *Dialysis is three times a week. I can't do that. I have to work!*
- *If I don't do dialysis, does that mean I am going to die?*
- *I have so many questions, and all the information is over-whelming to me!*

Journaling Questions

1. *What are my biggest fears right now?*
2. *My questions are…*

Information

- There are five stages of CKD. The stages are determined by blood work, specifically urine albumin and glomerular filtration rate (GFR).
- GFR is the flow rate of fluid being filtered through the kidney. It is a calculation based on age, gender, race, and a blood test.
- Stage 1 and 2 are typically asymptomatic. By stage 3, one can experience signs of anemia, decreased urine output, and swelling. By stage 4, usually a nephrologist has been consulted to provide guidance in preventing further deterioration of kidney function. If appropriate, a discussion of transplant may be initiated.
- Stage 5 requires kidney dialysis.
- Once a person reaches stage 5, their kidneys are working at about 10 percent.
- Dialysis is necessary when any of the following are experienced:
  - high potassium levels
  - shortness of breath caused by fluid buildup around the heart and lungs
  - uremia (toxins in the blood that the kidneys cannot clear)

- Some people have residual kidney function. This means they still produce urine, even near normal amounts, but their kidneys no longer filter out the toxins.
- The buildup of toxins can be fatal; therefore, dialysis is necessary to prevent death.
- Dialysis treatments are required three times per week, each lasting approximately four hours.
- Most dialysis units have three shifts to accommodate patients' schedules.
- Other options are available, such as nighttime dialysis, home dialysis, or peritoneal dialysis. Ask for more information about these options.
- Full-time work is possible if your schedule has flexibility.
- CKD is considered a permanent disability.
- The social worker will help you and your family navigate through your choices and help you to make decisions by providing the financial information and answer insurance/benefit questions.

Words of Comfort

The Lord is my shepherd, I lack nothing. He makes me lie down in green pastures, he leads me beside quiet waters, he refreshes my soul. He guides me along the right paths for his name's sake. Even though I walk through the darkest valley, I will fear no evil, for you are with me; your rod and your staff, they comfort me. You prepare a table before me in the presence of my enemies. You anoint my head with oil; my cup overflows. Surely your goodness and love will follow me all the days of my life, and I will dwell in the house of the Lord forever. (Psalm 23 NIV)

Gina Novak

Today's Prayer

    Lord, I need you now. I am scared and overwhelmed. Please comfort me in all my fears. Give me wisdom to ask the right questions. Help me to trust my providers. Give them compassion and understanding toward me. Strengthen my body and protect me from complications. Give me the courage to face medical procedures that may be uncomfortable.

Chapter 2

Reality Sets In

I can't believe this is happening. I now have a temporary dialysis catheter sticking out of my chest. It's ugly, sore, and even when I'm being careful, it seems to get tugged on. I'm not allowed to shower because of the risk of infection, and it gets even worse. I'm told that it is "temporary" only in the sense that I will need a more permanent method to receive dialysis. They gave me information about this, but all I can recall is that it means surgery.

Tomorrow I will be starting dialysis. I've been given an appointment at a dialysis clinic near my home. I'm barely even nervous because I've been feeling so poorly. I'm sick to my stomach all the time, but I've gained twelve pounds. My doctor tells me this is fluid, and that starting dialysis will help me to feel better.

Week 2

You now have a dialysis catheter in your chest and discussions have started regarding future surgery for a "permanent" method for dialysis. You may have noticed a worsening appetite, frequent nausea, and more swelling in your legs. It is difficult to make important decisions when you aren't feeling well. It may seem like you are just going through the motions without really understanding.

Journaling Questions

1. *How will I know if I am making the right medical decisions?*
2. *The questions I need answered now are?*

Information

- Dialysis catheters are inserted into a chest vein (subclavian) or neck vein (jugular) and tunneled under your skin. This is known as a cuffed catheter. The cuff acts as a barrier for preventing bacteria from entering the bloodstream.
- Catheters are invasive and, therefore, have an elevated risk of infection. For most individuals, catheters are considered a temporary access until a permanent one can be established. The goal for permanent access is within ninety days or less of your first dialysis treatment.
- Measures to prevent catheter infections are the following: no showering or swimming; avoid sleeping on or carrying items on the same side of the catheters location; wearing a button-down shirt during hemodialysis for easy access to the catheter; not removing the dressing between dialysis treatments; and notifying your dialysis team immediately if you develop fever, chills, or tenderness at the site. Only members of the dialysis team should use your catheter for drawing blood or giving fluids/medications.
- Catheters can develop fibrin clots. These clots are not blood clots, but they are problematic. They cause your catheter to function poorly.
- A poorly functioning catheter can be addressed in two ways. First, the nurse will attempt to restore function by giving a medication called Activase. It will dissolve the clot so that function can be restored.
- If the "clot-busting" medication, Activase, is not successful, then you may need to have a new catheter placed. This is a simple procedure done by an interventional radiologist. Sometimes it is referred to an "over-the-wire exchange." This means it is placed in the exact same spot.
- Your nephrology team will refer you to a vascular surgeon within the next few weeks. The surgeon will determine if you are suited best for a fistula or a graft.

- A fistula uses your native blood vessels by combining a vein and an artery. Fistulas have lesser rates of infection and clotting but require an eight- to twelve-week period of maturation before it can be used.
- A graft combines the artery and vein by use of a synthetic material. Grafts can be used within two to four weeks but have a slightly higher risk of infection and clotting than fistulas.
- Your vascular surgeon will make a recommendation of a fistula or a graft based on your medical history and by doing an ultrasound of your arms known as a vein mapping.
- Uremia (the buildup of toxins that your own kidneys can no longer filter) is the cause of your nausea and loss of appetite. The good news is that these symptoms will improve relatively quickly once dialysis has begun.
- The swelling and shortness of breath you are experiencing also will improve with dialysis. It may not resolve immediately as fluid cannot be removed all at once, but even within the first week of treatments, you should feel a noticeable difference.
- You are meeting many new people and being expected to trust the information they tell you. This is hard. You haven't had time to develop trust. Don't be afraid to ask questions over and over until you have a clear understanding of the information being given to you. Bring family/friends to hear the explanations as well.

Words of Comfort

Trust God from the bottom of your heart; don't try and figure out everything on your own. Listen for God's voice in everything you do, everywhere you go; he's the one who will keep you on track. (Proverbs 3:5–6 MSG)

Today's Prayer

Oh, mighty Father, I'm sick. I don't trust my own decisions and understanding. Help me to put my faith in you, Father. Provide me with all the right decisions about surgery. Bolster my faithfulness in you for protection. Keep me safe at dialysis tomorrow and take away this nausea and shortness of breath.

Chapter 3

What's Happening?

I've been to dialysis several times now. It's not easy, but I do feel phys-ically better, and that helps. The first time I saw my blood run through the tubing and back into my body was tough—I'm not kidding. It's also hard to sit among complete strangers while this is happening to my body. I feel so exposed, and yet the same thing is happening to everyone else too.

The staff are confident and capable; that helps too. I'm depending on them to do their job right; my life is at stake. This is a serious disease. I need surgery, blood work every couple of weeks, and to come to dialysis three times a week for the rest of my life. I'm being told a lot of informa-tion every treatment. I have met a dietician, social worker, nurse practi-tioner, technician, charge nurse, and the administrative assistant. Each person is teaching me something. I like that information gets repeated over and over. I feel like I'm starting to understand a little bit. I don't feel as scared as I did.

I also recognize the other patients on my shift. When my anxi-ety creeps in, like when my machine starts alarming, I look over at the patient across from me, and she just nods. She understands my fear. I wonder if she knows how very much this comforts me.

Week 3

By now, the uremia or toxins have been reduced through dial-ysis, and the nausea is gone. You feel a little more like your old self, perhaps ready to absorb more information. But then, whoa, how much are you expected to know? It's normal to need information reviewed and reviewed. Each provider comes with their own topic to teach. Also, you may be hearing unfamiliar words. Take it slow. You are not expected to know everything immediately. Learn from everybody. Write things down. Ask for reading materials to take home, websites, support groups. Talk to other patients to gain their understanding and perspective.

Journaling Question

The main questions that I need answered are?

Information

- The dialysis machine works by removing blood through the arterial side of your catheter, fistula, or graft, cleaning it through a *dialyzer* and returning it to your body in the venous portion of your catheter, fistula, or graft.
- The dialyzer is a tube filled with hollow straw-like membranes. Your blood goes through each of the hollow straws, and fluid goes around and between each straw. The blood and fluid *never* mix.
- The fluid is called *dialysate*. The exact chemical composition is prescribed by your nurse practitioner (NP) or nephrologist (MD). It is based on your blood chemistries. It contains calcium, potassium, dextrose, and magnesium.
- No more than 300ccs of blood is outside of your body at one given time. This is equal to about one and a quarter cup. The average adult has between one and one-half gallons of blood in the body.
- When blood is outside of your body and moving through the dialyzer, it can begin to clot. This is prevented by giving a small dose of a blood thinner with each treatment. The blood thinner is called heparin and only lasts for six hours.
- Each dialysis unit has a dietician. They will help you modify your diet to be kidney friendly, as well as provide tips about protein, fluid restriction, and hidden sources of

phosphorus. The dietician meets with you at least monthly. They can also help with food shopping, binder adherence, and recipes.

- Each dialysis unit has a social worker. They will assist you with insurance questions, applying for disability, determining what prescription program is best for you, and navigating the transportation assistance that is available to you. They also will assess for signs of anxiety, depression, and help you with coping skills as you transition to a lifestyle with CKD.
- Each dialysis unit is comprised of registered nurses and certified dialysis technicians. They are licensed and state registered. They are experts in working with the dialysis machines, water systems, and placing your needles for dialysis.
- Each dialysis unit has a variety of administrative personnel who will help you with paperwork, shift-change requests, traveling, and just about anything you may need.
- Finally, dialysis units are *not* staffed with physicians. A nephrologist will see you monthly at the dialysis unit. Some units are staffed with physician extenders such as nurse practitioners or physician assistants. All hemodialysis units must have a medical director who oversees all operations and policies related to patient care.

Words of Comfort

Do not be anxious about anything, but in every situation, by prayer and petition, with thanksgiving, present your requests to God. And the peace of God, which transcends all understanding, will guard your hearts and minds in Christ Jesus. (Philippians 4:6–7 NIV)

Today's Prayer

King of Kings, I lift to you all my anxieties. Lord, take away my fears when the machine beeps or my blood stops or other unexpected things occur. Lord, grant me your peace every day when I come to dialysis. Help me to not worry about what I don't know. Thank you for all the staff. Thank you for their knowledge and compassion in caring for me. Help me to believe in their skills and trust them completely.

Chapter 4

Thanks Be to Dialysis

Dialysis has been lifesaving for me. I was living on borrowed time before I started. I could barely walk ten feet without getting short of breath. I had gained forty pounds of fluid and diagnosed with congestive heart failure (CHF). My heart doctor said my heart function was so bad that I needed a defibrillator and lifelong blood thinners.

Then I came to the hemodialysis clinic. I figured anything would be better than my current situation. The staff told me I was unusual because I kept saying how much better I felt after each four-hour session. The staff told me once more fluid came off me, I would feel even better. They were right. I became so appreciative of these technicians and nurses. I rarely had any questions. Everything the staff did for me, I viewed it as a huge blessing. I put my trust in them completely, and I tried to express my gratitude every single day!

I became nicknamed the "poster child." I did just about everything they told me, and this resulted in improved blood work results. I was told they were near perfect. I was able to watch my boy play basketball again. I was even able to sit in the bleachers. My wife and I started to take walks, and she became invested in my healthcare. My marriage improved in many ways!

Maybe I am unique in how I think and feel about my treatments? As my health improved, so did my quality of life. I know for a fact that dialysis has increased the quantity of my days, and for this, I am forever thankful!

By the way, my heart failure has improved so much that my heart doctor said I know longer need a defibrillator, and I might become eligible for the transplant list.

Week 4

It is a good sign that you are feeling better with dialysis treatments. This negates those earlier doubts you had about, whether you really needed to start HD. The fact that you are no longer nauseated and having improved breathing are all indications of improved chemistry and fluid status within your body.

Also, by now, you have gained trust in these "strangers" from a few weeks ago. Just as you have become familiar with different staff members, they too have become familiarized with the nuances of your needs. You will naturally develop staff preferences and come to the reality that you will not always have the same people taking care of you. This is sometimes difficult as it is an important aspect of your care, and yet you have little control.

Journaling Question

Since I feel so much better, what are the limits of what I can do?

Information

- Many individuals begin dialysis extremely overloaded with fluid. These symptoms are shortness of breath when lying down or with exertion like walking.
- As fluid is removed each session, these symptoms should become noticeably improved.
- The key to reaching your ideal body weight (IBW) or target weight (TW) is to limit your fluid gains between each session. The recommended intradialytic weight gain (IDWG) is between two to three kilograms.
- Gaining greater than two to three kilograms between treatments makes it difficult to improve the symptoms mentioned above. Fluid restriction is generally set to thirty-two ounces daily.
- If you find yourself with an increased thirst and a need for more than thirty-two ounces daily, schedule a meeting with

the dietician. He/she will likely discover a high salt/sodium content in your current food choices and help you develop a plan to reduce this.

- As your fluid status improves, it is important to become more active. Your body will alert you when you are doing too much. For example, you may only be able to take a half of a flight of stairs before resting. This is perfectly okay. Keep track of your own progress in activity. Discuss with your providers what your activity goal is. Be specific!

- Congestive heart failure (CHF) is a combination of increased blood volume and a weakened heart muscle. The heart can no longer pump out enough volume, and so there is a decrease in oxygenated blood flow to your organs.

- CHF is common, but it is a serious condition. The heart muscle can become extremely weak. This is often diagnosed by a test known as an echocardiogram or an ultrasound of the heart.

- CHF can improve especially in the setting of volume overload. As the volume of fluid is reduced in your body, the demands on the heart are less.

- When the heart pump is extremely weak, your cardiologist may recommend blood thinners and an internal defibrillator. Discuss your concerns with your provider.

Words of Comfort

All things are possible with God. (Mark 10:27b NIV)

Today's Prayer

Lord God, thank you for restoring my breath, for making each day just a little easier to navigate. May all my days glorify your name and honor you. May I not be limited to my own thinking but count on your possibilities. Amen.

Chapter 5

Kindness Matters

Today one of my fellow patients celebrated her eighty-seventh birthday. I'm not exactly sure how long she has been on dialysis; she was here when I started four years ago. I've noticed that she is less talkative and now arrives in a wheelchair instead of using her walker as she once did. Her physical health seems to have declined, but I can tell that the staff adore her. They have pet names for her. They put her cushion under her the way she is most comfortable. They sit with her and hold her sites because she no longer has the strength to hold her own sites. I appreciate watching this kindness: it makes me feel safe and protected.

Today the kindness shown was extra special. It was about midtreatment when a group of our hardworking technicians gathered around her. They sang and danced a special birthday wish. They also presented her with a pink sprinkled doughnut! The surprised smile on this elderly lady's face was beautiful. The moment was beautiful!

Week 5

You may have started to notice by this point that you are more relaxed at your sessions. You still have a great deal to learn about your illness and the treatment, but you may have noticed that you have a less frantic or anxious attachment to the learning. You are able to look beyond your own needs and realize that observation of others is a great way to learn.

The routine of the dialysis flow may now feel familiar. You know more of what is to be expected, what issues can occur in the unit, and specific care needs of your fellow "dialysis mates." You may begin friendships or at least enough familiarity with others that it feels safe to share some of your questions, concerns, and/or experiences.

A kinship or family-like environment does typically develop within your "shift." You notice when someone is missing. You may even voice your concerns to the staff about individuals. In the waiting room, you may be able to match family members with patients and know who rides with who and who lives near who. Ideally, you also have started to recognize how staff members are invested and concerned for those they care for. Care beyond the basic needs, but in a way that shows you they know their patients' story, their lives have touched one another and a bond beyond what you expected, exists.

Journaling Questions

1. *Is this a safe environment for me to invest in? What do I feel comfortable sharing?*
2. *How might I invest in others? What do I have to offer?*

Information

- Pressure must be applied to your sites when the needle is removed. Standard policy states that one needle is removed at a time, and pressure is applied for approximately five minutes.
- Everyone is taught how to don a glove and apply direct pressure over their sites.
- Some circumstances prevent an individual from being able to do this. Examples are someone who has had a stroke and sustained hand weakness, some elderly or others suffering with other illnesses in addition to CKD.
- Once the bleeding stops, a dressing is applied. This varies by unit policy but usually consists of a gauze and tape or a Band-Aid.
- The dressings should be removed after four hours as prolonged pressure can compromise the blood flow and cause the access to clot off.

- Prolonged bleeding (greater than fifteen minutes) after the needle has been removed may indicate that there is a narrowing of the vessel above the site, or that your blood thinner dose needs adjusted, or the placement of your fingers were not directly over the site. The staff will help determine this and take the needed course of action.
- The staff will come to know your individual preferences, which needle you like pulled first, how you like your bandage applied, etc.
- The staff also will also come to know your *comfort* preferences during your treatment such as if you prefer the TV or listen to your own music, the position of your chair, where your belongings are placed in proximity to your reach, blanket/pillow or not, chair heater and massager on or off.
- Your comfort is important to you and the staff. Ask for those things that make a difference for you. This is especially important if there is substitute staff working or if it has been a particularly busy day.
- When a staff forgets your needs, it's not out of lack of concern but rather other priorities pressing on their workflow. Just ask for the things you need.
- How much or how little you share about your personal life is *entirely* up to you. Do what feels most comfortable to you.
- The average length of dialysis is five years, but this does vary greatly. Three times per week at four hours per session multiplied by five years equals 3,120 hours! That is a lot of time to get to know someone!

Words of Comfort

> Truly I tell you, whatever you did for one of
> the least of these brothers and sisters of mine, you
> did for me. (Matthew 25:40 NIV)

Today's Prayer

Father, help me to remember that in the end, only kindness matters. Let my words, my body language, and my actions toward my brother show kindness always. Help me to remember that when my needs are feeling neglected or overlooked by others, that it is not intentional but rather human. Let me show grace to all who care for me and my friends.

Chapter 6

Sometimes Tears Fall

At any given time, tears will fall among us patients during treatment time. Sometimes the reasons aren't known; sometimes they are because of pain from cramping.

I have chronic obstructive pulmonary disease (COPD) in addition to my CKD. It makes my breathing a challenge every single day. When I come to dialysis short of breath, it is hard to tell if it is from too much fluid, another lung infection, or if I am just so tired from working so hard to breathe for so long. I have days when it is too much. I know my health is very poor. I've discussed it with my doctors, my family, and my God.

Today was a day when it felt too hard. I was miserable, and I honestly didn't know what I wanted. I derived at the decision to stop my treatment an hour early. In fact, I insisted! I became loud, and my breathing worsened from expending this extra energy. Suddenly, I was in that desperate place again.

And then the unexpected happened. A staff member knelt beside me, her eyes filled with competence and confidence that this wasn't my end. Her eyes more importantly told me she cared. She touched my hand ever so gently as I was crying, "God, help me. I can't breathe." As my tears fell, her eyes filled with similar tears, and she said, "I know you are a woman of faith, so I feel like I can share this with you. When I have desperation set in, I am comforted that he knows every one of my tears. He counts them and places them in his bottle. It reminds me that I am not alone." Then she said to me, "And you are not alone."

Week 6

Living with dialysis brings an unpredictable aspect to life. One moment, you may feel fine like you don't even have kidney disease! The next, you may feel you don't have the energy to go through it for one more moment. It can be frustrating, especially when you have done all the things you have been told, and then out of the blue, *bam!* You're not doing so well. Not only is this frustrating and scary for you, it is equally disconcerting to your loved ones who are trying to watch over you and make sure you stay on track.

Journaling Questions

1. *How can I better cope with all the unknowns of this disease?*
2. *Are there any resources available to my family?*

Information

- Shortness of breath (SOB) is an extremely frightening experience. It is normal to feel panicky and desperate if this occurs.
- If your respirations are rapid, you feel dizzy, palpitations, and/or perspiring, call 911.
- Severe shortness of breath with the symptoms noted above can quickly deteriorate into pulmonary edema (fluid in the lungs). This can be life-threatening and needs to be addressed quickly rather than waiting for the next dialysis treatment.
- If you develop an acute onset of SOB, call 911, elevate the head of your bed or sit forward, slow your breathing through pursed lips, and do your best to stay calm.
- If this occurs at the dialysis center, oxygen will be administered as well, your oxygen level will be checked with a pulse oximeter, and extra fluid will be removed. The nurse's assessment will determine if you can be safely dialyzed in the dialysis unit. If you are unstable, you will be transported

to the hospital by the emergency medical system (EMS). Symptoms indicating that you are unstable are chest pain, worsening of your breathing, and extreme blood pressure and heart rate readings.

- Dialysis in the ER is not immediately available. Therefore, if you are stable, it is in your best interest to be dialyzed at the center.
- Tips for avoiding large fluctuations in your fluid gains include adhering to your prescribed fluid restriction (usually two to three kilogram weight gain between treatments is acceptable).
- Before each treatment, you are weighed by one of the staff members. This is called your pre-weight. Obtaining accurate weights is of the utmost importance.
- Ensuring an accurate pre-weight can be done by making sure the scale is zeroed before stepping on, standing still in the center of the scale, removing all items from your pockets, and removing heavy coats/shoes/or jewelry
- If your pre-weight seems unusually low (minimal fluid gain), recheck your weight! Having a falsely low reading will result in an insufficient fluid amount to be removed. This increases the likelihood of fluid overload.
- If your pre-weight seems unusually *high*, double-check your weight. Having a falsely high reading will result in too much fluid removal leading to cramps, dizziness, nausea, and perhaps fainting.
- As the weather changes, your clothing weight will too. Summer means lighter clothing, and your TW will need to be reduced. Cooler weather means heavier clothing, and your TW will need to be increased.
- An intake of high sodium foods will increase your fluid gains, even if it is just one meal.
- Restaurant and fast foods will always have a higher salt content than home-cooked meals.
- Foods to avoid are soups, Chinese food, chips/salted pretzels, snack foods like Pringles, Fritos, Doritos, etc.

- Every dialysis unit has a full-time social worker available to you and your family. This individual is prepared to help you with coping skills during this adjustment period and is also readily available to your significant others. He/she can answer many of your questions and can refer you to available resources.
- Crying is a coping mechanism for fear, anger, frustration, and many other emotions.

Words of Comfort

You've kept track of my every toss and turn through the sleepless nights, Each tear entered in your ledger, each ache written in your book. (Psalm 56:8 MSG)

Today's Prayer

Lord, soothe my worry, my hurt. I cannot bear this pain without you by my side. Bring me comfort through my caretakers. Give them the competence and skill to meet my needs. Bring comfort to my family and ease their fears and their tears. Bolster us with the courage that can only come from your strength. Amen.

Chapter 7

I Care for You, and I Care about You

Sometimes my frustration shows up in my tone and in my body language when you show up late, leave early, or come in volume overloaded. You may think that I have "attitude" because I don't like my job, but the truth is…I love my job and care deeply about your well-being. When you show up late or leave early, I can't provide you with the care you need. Even more frustrating is when you come with way too much fluid on. Not only are you miserable because you can't breathe, but it scares me knowing how risky this is for your life. Honestly, sometimes it feels like I care more for your life than you do.

Week 7

As you are adjusting to dialysis, it may seem as though you have acquired a great deal of *bosses*. I am speaking of the staff. They give you numerous directives each time you come, "get your weight," "you are sitting in this chair today," "you are late, you won't receive your full treatment today." These statements can be a matter-of-fact and with little explanation. Time efficiency at the dialysis center is necessary to accommodate the three, sometimes four, shifts of patients that receive dialysis each day.

You may have been the recipient of other comments that seem harsh and uncaring. Statements like, "You are drinking too much fluid. We can't take it all off!"

On the surface, it may seem like their words are unkind, without compassion, like they don't understand how difficult this all is.

If these are the conclusions you have made about the staff, they are inaccurate. Read the facts below for further understanding.

Journaling Questions

1. *How come some of the staff seem so unfriendly toward me?*
2. *How should I react to their brisk words and attitude?*

Information

- Dialysis is provided by certified dialysis technicians.
- Technicians are high school/or equivalent graduates who are trained and certified and receive intensive on-the-job training provided by a dialysis company.
- Dialysis nurses are registered and state licensed who require intense on-the-job training provided by a dialysis company.
- RNs may not be in charge until six months to one year from their hire date.
- All staff are trained and tested in many areas (water systems, set up and working of dialysis machines, cannulation, programming of machines, documentation, etc.).
- Dialysis technicians and nurses use their experience to assure your treatments are safe and effective.
- Policies guide decisions regarding the amount of fluid that can be removed in one dialysis session.
- Years of experience and their knowledge of their patients further enhance the care they provide.
- Dialysis units typically run three shifts of patients.
- Dialysis staff arrive early in the am to set up and prepare for patient care.
- Dialysis staff typically work twelve to fourteen hours per day.
- Dialysis staff are trained to independently act on critical situations such as fluid resuscitation, bleeding emergencies, and seizures. Their immediate assessments and actions of the patients save lives!

- Dialysis staff are invested in their careers but more importantly invested in you!
- Efficiency and competence are necessary to provide safe care to *all*.
- Centers for Medicaid and Medicare Services (CMS) currently recommends that no more than thirteen cubic centimeters per kilogram per hour of fluid be removed during dialysis. This recommendation stems from suspected cardiac ramifications with chronic high volume removal. Providers can override this restriction, but staff cannot independently override this regulation without an order.
- The fluid removal restriction means that you can only remove between three to five kilograms in each treatment. The smaller your body size, the less fluid you will be able to remove safely according to the CMS recommendation.
- Shortened dialysis time, missed treatments, or failure to restrict your fluid gains between dialysis sessions will all put you at a greater risk for fluid overload, also known as hypervolemia.
- Signs/symptoms of hypervolemia include shortness of breath, elevated weight, swelling, elevated blood pressure, and an elevated pulse rate.
- Hypervolemia is one of the leading causes of emergency room visits, hospitalizations, and death in dialysis patients.
- A general rule of thumb is to limit your fluid intake to thirty-two ounces daily and an inter-dialytic weight gain between sessions of two to three liters.

Words of Comfort

So in everything, do to others what you would have them do to you, for this sums up the Law and the Prophets. (Matthew 7:12 NIV)

Today's Prayer

Oh, mighty Maker of all things, do not let me misinterpret the care given to me by others. Help me to know that they are for me and not against me and are here to provide me with important information and safe care. Forgive me when I doubt, when I fear, when I myself am unkind in word and action. Lord, give me self-control in my fluid intake and guard my sharp tongue when I become frustrated. Amen.

Chapter 8

My Past Doesn't Dictate My Future

I am a kidney dialysis patient. I mistreated my body for years when I was a younger man. I was stubborn, I didn't listen to medical advice, and I acted like I was invincible. It eventually caught up with me. I fought it a few more years, doing things "my way."

Now I look back and realize all the harsh truths given to me by my doctors were because they cared. Now I come to dialysis treatments three times every week—nine years and counting. My body does okay, but my past did not leave me without reminders. I have significant bone disease and require expensive medicines to treat it. I am getting older too, so other medical conditions have appeared. I had to have back surgeries and dental work.

But here is the thing, I acknowledge that my stubbornness and poor decisions from my past do not dictate my future. I am a "stellar" patient now. I never miss treatments, even when I go out of town. I was asked by the clinic to advocate for the patients on my treatment days by attending monthly meetings with the care team. I have been invited by my doctor to speak at Grand Rounds on multiple occasions. I even wrote an article for our Clinic's newsletter!

I am not a churchgoing kind of guy, even though my father is a pastor. But I do know that we get second, third, and more chances in life. I am so grateful that there were MDs, RNs, technicians, and my own wonderful loving family who never gave up on me. This support has been life-changing and life-saving for me. Hallelujah!

Week 9

As you glance across the room and see other patients who seem to have it all together, trust me in this, their story too had bumps along the way. The journey of a chronic illness such as kidney disease is a process. Although it is true that some people accept the diagnosis and adapt quickly to this life change, most do not!

Most people, perhaps you, fight the process every step of the way. Most people take a full one year to accept the new realities of the diagnosis and treatment. Sadly, some resist the necessary adjustments even up until their last breath.

Journaling Questions

1. *What changes in my lifestyle are required right now?*
2. *What changes in my life will be required for the long run?*

Information

- The most common causes for needing dialysis is high blood pressure that has been poorly controlled, and diabetes that has been poorly controlled.
- High blood pressure, called hypertension, is typically a silent illness and, therefore, often mistakenly ignored.
- Hypertension requires lifestyle modifications in diet and weight, as well as strict adherence to lifelong medications.
- Diabetes requires diligence with diet, medications, and follow-up care.
- "Pretty good control" of one's sugar does not prevent the macro- and microvascular changes that occur within your blood vessels and organs.
- Once irreversible changes occur resulting in CKD-5, HTN and diabetes control will still be of extreme importance. Controlling this disease will not result in restored kidney function but rather prevent further injuries to your heart, eyes, lungs, and vascular systems.

- Bone disease is a consequence of CKD-5 and results from an imbalance in calcium and phosphorus levels.
- Healthy bones need calcitriol (the active form of vitamin D), which is made in the kidney. Calcitriol maintains your blood calcium level and promotes bone formation.
- Our kidneys also remove phosphorus from our blood, which we acquire through the foods we eat.
- Additionally, the parathyroid glands (four located in your neck) regulate calcium in your blood by the hormone PTH.
- PTH regulates the calcium in your blood by moving it from your bones. It restores the balance in your blood but starves the bones of calcium.
- The result of *poorly controlled calcium, phosphorus, and PTH* is weak bones producing bone and joint pain and calcifications in the blood vessels and heart.
- These three blood tests are monitored closely and discussed with you every month.
- Based on your blood results, adjustments may be recommended in your diet and medications.

Words of Comfort

> If you, Lord, kept a record of sins, Lord who could stand? (Psalm 130:3 NIV)

Today's Prayer

Lord, you know all my past mistakes, my bad choices, and how I've ignored my own health. For this, I confess and invite your healing Spirit into my presence. Give me strength and courage to face my current situation. I am comforted by knowing you will never turn away from me. You are my rock and my salvation. Amen.

Chapter 9

What if I Cannot Do This?

I look around at the other patients and just know that there are some things I cannot do. I see Mr. A who has large bumps on his arms; they're called aneurysms. My gut reaction to this is repulsion. I cannot allow this to happen to my body.

Then I look over at Mrs. G. She is an older woman who bleeds for long times after her needles are removed. I can't tell you how many times she has been sent to the hospital after dialysis because they can't stop the bleeding. She begs them to let her go home as the staff explain why this is not safe. I feel so sorry for her, all the while thinking. I hope that never happens to me.

And Mr. M., his treatments start before me and end after me. He has five-hour treatments compared to my three. "Five hours, no way will I do that."

Week 9

With thirty dialysis sessions under your belt, you may now be able to focus on your surroundings. This will include the other patients around you. Most dialysis centers are set up with chairs that are close to one another. The people on either side of you become your neighbors. Despite efforts to maintain confidentiality, you will learn private information about them, and they will learn about you. There is comfort and camaraderie that develops. Patients become encouragers to one another. Likewise, when one of your comrades suffers, you will carry their pain. It is not unusual to feel deep compassion and even grief when you observe suffering in one of your newly acquired family members.

You may observe the experiences of others and hope that this never happens to you. Some of the circumstances related to dialysis are incredibly challenging. It is completely understandable for these thoughts to enter your mind and even cause you some degree of worry.

Journaling Questions

1. *Can I have time to think about the tough decisions regarding the recommendations of my care?*
2. *When I see "my neighbors" struggle, how can I best encourage them?*

Information

- Aneurysms occur when areas of the fistula develop wall weakening, resulting in dilations that look like *bumps*.
- Aneurysms are best prevented by rotation of the needle sites.
- Aneurysms are dangerous if the overlying skin becomes shiny and thin or if the width doubles to two and a half times the normal width.
- Large or concerning aneurysms can usually be surgically repaired with minimal to no disruption in your treatments, but this does require vascular surgery.
- Once the needles are removed, the area should bleed no longer than fifteen minutes.
- Prolonged bleeding can be a sign of a narrowing of the access above the needle site called stenosis. The back pressure upstream can cause more forceful bleeding.
- Prolonged bleeding can also occur when someone takes blood thinners, is receiving large amounts of heparin with dialysis, has a low platelet count, or improperly holds pressure over the sites after the needles are removed.

- The staff will assist you with donning a glove and place your finger properly over the needle site when your treatment is finished.
- Some patients will require assistance holding their sites, or perhaps clamps will be applied.
- Duration of dialysis treatments are determined by your nephrology provider. Considerations to determine the time needed are your body surface area (weight/height), your access type, and your blood test results.
- In general, shorter treatment times are inadequate to clear one's body of middle molecule toxins that are not measurable. The standard of practice currently recommends starting new patients at three and a half hours, thrice weekly.
- It is not unusual to need more dialysis time as the years pass. Residual renal function naturally declines, and unfortunately, there is no exact measures to prevent this decline.
- Your treatment plan is individualized by your provider. All concerns should always be discussed so that you have all the necessary information to make good decisions regarding your care.
- Maintaining your privacy is important. If you are concerned about compromising yours, ask for a private meeting to discuss your care. This is very doable but not routinely offered due to the time constraints. Meetings can be completed using telemedicine, scheduled group conferences, or one-on-one meetings.

Words of Comfort

No temptation or test that comes your way is beyond the course of what others have had to face. All you need to remember is that God will never let you down; he'll never let you be pushed past your limit; he'll always be there to help you come through it. (1 Corinthians 10:13 MSG)

Gina Novak

Today's Prayer

God, I need you here in this dialysis unit every single moment. So much goes on here that is beyond my comprehension. I know you are in control. I pray for the safekeeping of my neighbors. I pray for my own worries. You know me better than I know myself. I am faithful that you will not give me more than I can handle. I am faithful you will hold me up when I cannot stand alone. Amen.

Chapter 10

I've Got This!

I'm not the typical dialysis patient. First, I'm young (thirty-two). I still work full-time. I've got people who rely on me. I can't just not show up for them. I've missed dialysis treatments plenty of times; my body handles it fine. I know my body and what I can handle.

I get so annoyed with the staff with their lectures about skipping treatments. My labs are good, so what's the problem? I tell them that I appreciate their concern. I listen to their well-meaning advice. But honestly, I would prefer that they would leave me alone.

Don't get me wrong. I appreciate everything the staff does. I know they work hard, and for most patients, their input is necessary. But I'm different. I know when I need dialysis, I wish that I could get them to understand this.

Week 10

Some patients can miss treatments without immediate untoward complications, especially when first diagnosed with stage 5 CKD. To be clear, complications and risks are two different subjects. Each time a dialysis session is missed, a risk for death exists. Hyperkalemia (an elevated potassium) can cause an irregular and fatal heart rhythm. This is fact. Does it happen every time a patient skips a treatment? No. Is the risk present? Yes!

The reason that some patients are falsely lured into believing that skipping treatments is a safe practice is because they are in denial. Healthy kidneys function twenty-four hours a day, seven days a week, or 168 hours every single week. A typical dialysis week provides twelve hours of filtering and cleaning the blood. Lowering this by any number has a cascading effect not limited to the buildup of toxins, which can have a ripple effect on the heart, lungs, gut, and immune system. Additionally, each time a person chooses to skip a treatment, they are also missing medications prescribed with each treatment. These medications are necessary to prevent anemia, iron deficiency, bone disease, and secondary hyperparathyroidism (SHPT).

Adjustment to a newly diagnosed chronic illness and the required life change is difficult. Denial can be a common part of the adjustment process.

Denial of your illness can be reinforced when it appears that you've "gotten away" with skipping a treatment. The staff are well aware of this slippery slope of thinking and, therefore, will confront you regarding your attendance by presenting you with facts of the associated dangers.

Journaling Questions

1. *How come I feel fine when I miss treatments?*
2. *Why can't I try less time or less days?*

Information

- Standard of care for stage 5 CKD in the United States is dialysis three times per week.
- Standard dialysis sessions are between three hours to five hours. The duration is determined by body size, fluid to be removed, access adequacy, and other diseases present.
- The most common complication associated with a missed dialysis session is hypervolemia or too much fluid.
- Hypervolemia symptoms include shortness of breath, hypertension, swelling, pulmonary edema, and respiratory failure.
- The dialysis machine removes fluid, potassium, and calcium determined by the prescription written by your provider.

- Other elements managed by the dialysis machine are acidity, middle molecules, and other less measurable known toxins.
- Medications are often administered during dialysis treatments. Some are administered with each treatment, and some are less frequent.
- Erythrocyte stimulating agents (ESAs) are commonly administered. They stimulate the bone marrow to produce red blood cells necessary to prevent anemia.
- Vitamin D analogues are another commonly administered drug. The kidneys normally produce vitamin D, but this is reduced with CKD stage 5 leading to bone disease.
- Both ESAs and Vitamin D analogues cannot be *doubled* to make up for missed doses. Therefore, missed doses will impact your risks of anemia and bone disease.
- Dialysis requires lifestyle adjustments for you and your family. It is difficult to accept as a permanent part of your current life, and it is important to recognize this difficulty.
- Resistance to the adjustment is not uncommon. The staff are ready to help you field your questions and your emotions.
- All dialysis units are staffed with a full-time social worker who can help you process any additional needs you may have at this time. (Work options, financial/insurance questions, and assessing for depression and referring you to available resources.)
- Skipping a treatment does not necessarily mean you will end of up in the hospital. However, statistics show that your risk is much higher by doing so.
- Hypervolemia, the main reason for skipped treatment associated ER visits, can require high flow oxygen, CPAP-forced air into your lungs through a mask, and even intubation and artificial ventilation.
- Missed treatments almost always result in hypertension.
- Missed treatment due to feeling ill on the day of your scheduled treatment is different than an intentional skip-

ping but still often results in the complications previously mentioned.

- It is in your best interest to schedule a makeup treatment so that you still get three treatments per week.

Words of Comfort

> Take good counsel and accept correction that's the way to live wisely and well. (Proverbs 19:20 MSG)

Today's Prayer

Holy Father, I beg you to control my will. I know I must accept that dialysis is a necessary part of my life. As much as I know this, I want it not to be so. Amen.

Chapter 11

I Am So Very Tired!

Fatigue doesn't even begin to explain how I feel. I am dead-bone tired, lack of energy for everything; even cleaning up and getting dressed takes effort. I think I'm hungry, but, oh, the energy of deciding what is safe to eat and then trying to prepare it differently than I have after all these years. I'll just skip it and have a snack if I'm hungry!

Week 11

So you are three months into dialysis at this point; a great deal has happened. The seriousness of the disease has likely made its impact including frequent blood work, additional procedures or surgeries, and the wear and tear of going to dialysis treatments three times every week.

In addition to the abundant amount of new information you have received, you may have experienced contradictory information. There also is the emotional stress of learning to trust *strangers* and knowing your life depends on them doing their job properly.

Fatigue is part of the transition phase to dialysis. Knowing that this is part of the natural process can alleviate "unnecessary worry" that you may be experiencing.

Journaling Questions

1. *Are there any suggestions for coping with my low level of energy?*
2. *Do I need to consider medication for stress or insomnia?*

Information

- If you started dialysis using a catheter by the three-month mark, you should be ready to use your fistula or graft.
- Having your catheter removed is a tremendous accomplishment and one that immediately improves your survival rate, as well as decreases your risk for infection.
- Once you begin using your fistula (AVF) or graft (AVG), your treatment times may take a little longer due to cannulation and bleeding times.
- Fatigue is multifactorial, anemia associated with CKD, large volume removal, poor nutrition, and poor sleep hygiene are just a few of the contributors.
- A multivitamin may be prescribed. Most vitamins are not covered by standard prescription coverage. Special programs may be available to assist you with this expense depending on the state you live in and your income. Talk to your social worker about available resources.
- Do not purchase over-the-counter (OTC) vitamins without first consulting your dietician as some products contain magnesium, calcium, and other elements that must be restricted in CKD.
- Anemia secondary to lack of erythropoietin, produced by the kidneys, is a very common problem in CKD. This can be managed very effectively by iron and medications administered during dialysis. Standard care involves checking your hemoglobin levels monthly or more frequently.
- Iron deficiency can contribute to anemia. Your iron stores are checked monthly when on HD. Your provider may prescribe an iron supplement at home or prescribe intravenous iron to be given at the HD center.
- Oral iron supplements are not well absorbed and can cause gastrointestinal upset. If this is your experience, be sure to ask your provider for other options.

- Intravenous iron is usually well tolerated. Some experience a metallic taste when receiving intravenous iron. This rapidly resolves and still is reported to be preferable to oral supplementation by most HD patients.
- Poor nutritional intake is also a common concern both before and during dialysis. All HD units have dieticians on staff for guiding patients on proper intake and tips on addressing protein sources.
- Sleep hygiene should be addressed between you and your provider, although long-term sleeping/anxiety medication is *not* recommended. Short-term medication may be appropriate for extreme situations.
- Limiting inter-dialytic weight gains (IDWGs) to two to three kilograms will minimize the fluid and electrolyte shifts that can contribute to cramping and after treatment fatigue.
- Adequate protein intake is key to improving your immune system. Unlike CKD stage 4, once on dialysis, there is *no* protein restriction.
- Eggs, fish, chicken, and supplements are all acceptable sources of protein when on dialysis.
- Ideally, the goal for serum albumin is above four milligram per deciliter. Most centers have algorithms for oral nutrition supplementation. It may be a protein bar or drink given during dialysis to help boost one's levels.

Words of Comfort

Yet this I call to mind and therefore I have hope: Because of the Lord's great love we are not consumed, for his compassions never fail. They are new every morning; great is your faithfulness. (Lamentations 3:21–23 NIV)

Gina Novak

Today's Prayer

Lord, sustain me even when I feel too weak to go on. Give me the stamina to keep on keeping on. I know by your strength, I can do all things. Rest me when I am weary. Nourish me when I am weak. For it is not by my own power but yours that gives me the strength to face each day. Amen.

Chapter 12

Help Me, I'm Hurting

I had my fistula placed yesterday. It was done as an outpatient surgery. My arm is swollen and tender to touch. I was told to take the dressing off tomorrow and have the dialysis staff look at it. They felt around, listened to my arm with their stethoscope, and told me it was good. It doesn't feel good, but I have had worse pain in my life.

Just as I was thinking that thought, I developed the worst "charley horse" of my life. My calf muscle was tight and throbbing so much I screamed out help! My technician rushed to my side, followed closely behind by the nurse, and they gave me fluid through the machine. They also instructed me to flex my foot, but I couldn't. Finally, the technician picked up my leg and pushed my foot up toward my head and relief quickly followed. I was angry, scared, and grateful all at the same time. I felt beat-up and defeated. Now my arm and my leg were tender.

I thought dialysis was going to make me feel better.

Week 12

Although your access surgery was done as an outpatient procedure, it still involved surgery. Your suture line may be tender for a few days, and you will be given more information on how to care for it. Congratulations for doing one of the best things you can for yourself! Establishing a permanent access is one step closer to having your catheter removed, which reduces your risk of infection and other complications.

You also have experienced your first *cramp*. This is not pleasant. Every patient on dialysis has or will likely endure this in their dialysis experience. It likely indicates that you no longer have an excess of fluid buildup in your body.

It is quite normal to feel as though dialysis discomforts are too much for you to handle. This is particularly true at the beginning. You may even feel like it's not worth the torture, that you would rather take your chances without dialysis.

Journaling Questions

> *1. Is dialysis going to hurt?*
> *2. What should I expect to happen so I can be prepared?*

Information

- Both fistulas and grafts are placed in your nondominant arm most of the time.
- The day after surgery, it is normal for your arm and hand and possibly your fingers to be swollen.
- The dressing can be removed the very next day. Your incision can be washed with soap and water.
- If you have a great deal of swelling, some clear fluid may leak from the suture line. A small dressing or Band-Aid can be placed over these areas. It is not cause for alarm.
- Pain is best managed with elevating your arm on a pillow. You may take the prescribed pain medicine for a few days if the pain is moderate to severe. Tylenol can be used for milder pain.
- Remember all narcotics cause constipation, so prolonged use may require you to take a stool softener as well.
- The staff will listen and feel the access to determine if it is working properly. The sound heard is called a *bruit*, and the vibration felt is called a *thrill*.
- As your access matures, you will be taught how to feel or listen to your access.

- Muscle cramps at dialysis mean that fluid is being removed too quickly, *or* that you have reached your *target weight*, sometimes called *dry weight*.
- Target weight or dry weight is the amount you weigh with no extra fluid.
- At each dialysis session, you are required to get your weight before treatment. This is called *pre-weight*. Your established dry weight is subtracted from the pre-weight, and this is the amount of fluid your machine will be set to remove.
- Your dry weight is determined by your staff, but you too will learn how to decide how much fluid you can remove at one time.
- The standard is to remove less than one and a half liters per hour. Some patients tolerate much less than this. Some centers use a calculation of thirteen milliliters per kilogram per hour. Your provider will address the maximal safe amount for you. The numbers above are given as guidelines only.
- Once your dry weight is established, it may need changed from time to time.
- Obtaining accurate weights are *very* important to prevent cramping. Do not weigh with keys in your pocket or wearing a jacket or heavy shoes.
- If any weight obtained seems out of the ordinary, discuss with your technician to determine the correct amount to pull.

Words of Comfort

We are hard pressed on every side, but not crushed; perplexed, but not in despair; persecuted, but not abandoned; struck down, but not destroyed. (2 Corinthians 4:8 NIV)

Today's Prayer

Jesus, help me when I feel so desperate. I just want to give up. Let me remember that you are with me in the painful moments just as you have been present in the healthier times of my life. Help me to remember the experience of you in my life's trials and lift me up from these moments of despair. Comfort me when my pain is great, for you are greater. Amen.

Chapter 13

An Ordinary Day at the Market

I've learned to make the most of my non-dialysis days. Sometimes I am just too tired to do much of anything. On those days, I just forgive myself and rest. However, there are days when I feel more energy and desire to just go out and have an ordinary day. This may include a trip to the market, a walk through the mall, or a little walk down to the corner and back. Trust me, on the days, I feel normal, I want to make the most of them! Which is why this day—an ordinary day at the market—was so disappointing.

Being hungry with CKD is a challenge, but grocery shopping with CKD is the ultimate challenge. I learned to shop on the perimeter of the store where it is easier to stay away from packaged foods laden with salt, preservatives, and phosphate.

Can I just say that the perimeter of my store did not whet my appetite? In fact, I reached the checkout counter with nothing appealing and a heart full of heavy, wondering, "Is there anything good that I can have?"

Week 13

Dialysis serves to remove toxins from the bloodstream that are normally filtered by functioning kidneys. Unfortunately, not all electrolytes and molecules are filtered, as well as with healthy kidneys. This results in the need to adhere to certain dietary restrictions, as well as to take medications with each meal.

The renal diet is restrictive, and the phosphate binders taken with meals can cause gastrointestinal upset. It can make meal planning burdensome and eating a chore.

Each month, the dietician will review your labs, paying attention to things like potassium, calcium, phosphorus, and protein. He/she will also review your binders. Although the dietician is knowledgeable and helpful, the monthly lab review can feel like getting the results of a test, one that you tried your best on but did not score so well!

Journaling Questions

1. *How do I learn to adhere to a lifetime of dietary restrictions and still enjoy eating?*
2. *Can I ever eat out? How about special events like weddings, birthdays, and picnics?*
3. *What is some quick go-to foods that are good for me, appealing, and take little effort to prepare?*

Information

- Eating during dialysis treatments is not allowed due to the dangers of becoming hypotensive (dropping of blood pressure) and potentially choking.
- Blood shunting to the stomach can occur with a large intake of food, causing less blood flow to the brain and other organs, resulting in a drop in blood pressure and fainting.
- Most dialysis facilities will allow a sandwich-sized bag of appropriate snacks during treatment.
- Blood protein levels, known as albumin, is monitored monthly. Data has shown that HD patients have greater life expectancy when the albumin level is >4.0.
- The dietician and staff will provide you with a list of foods high in protein. These foods include eggs, fish, chicken, broccoli, and some protein bars.
- Phosphorus intake is the major challenge for dialysis patients.

- Phosphorus is contained in *many* foods. Examples are dried beans, red meats, chocolate, peanut butter, dark sodas, nuts, and dairy products to name a few.
- Reading food labels are key to knowing if your food contains phosphorous additives. Look for the following ingredients:
    o dicalcium phosphate
    o disodium phosphate
    o monosodium phosphate
    o phosphoric acid
    o sodium hexametaphosphate
    o trisodium phosphate
    o sodium tripolyphosphate
    o tetrasodium pyrophosphate

- Kidney-friendly recipes and meal plans are readily available on websites such as www.nkf.org.
- Phosphorus levels are monitored monthly with the desired range of 3.5–5.5 milligrams per deciliter.
- Potassium and sodium (salt) restrictions will be addressed in a later segment.
- Eating-out at restaurants or fast-food chains also requires some conscious choices. Fast-food options are usually salt laden and a poor choice. However, everyone is sometimes forced to use this option. Sodium content is readily available at most chains either on the menus or via the Internet. Do your homework.
- Restaurants also list sodium content. Using a search engine is easy to find information on most foods.
- Changing your habit by looking for heart-friendly or vegetarian options can also help you to avoid high salt content foods.
- Your dietician is an excellent resource. He/she will be able to help you with healthier substitutions for specific foods deemed not renal friendly.

Words of Comfort

> Therefore I tell you, do not worry about your life, what you will eat or drink; or about your body, what you will wear. Is not life more than food, and the body more than clothes? (Matthew 6:25 NIV)

Today's Prayer

Lord, take away my frustration about what I can and cannot eat. Give me the right amount of self-discipline when I am feeling discouraged and irritated over my disease restrictions. Help me to always have a thankful heart, to be grateful for life and not be so concerned with my eating habits. I lift this battle to you, Lord. Amen.

Chapter 14

When Is Enough Enough?

My mom has been on dialysis for nine years. Lately I feel like I am literally forcing her to go to her treatments. She says she is so tired and wants to skip just today? But this is becoming her story every morning. I hate waking her at three thirty in the morning and cajoling her into getting dressed and eating a little something before the van comes. It's especially hard when it is a rainy or cold morning. I feel cruel. The flip side to this is how awful it is to see her after she has skipped a treatment. She must fight for her air and barely can talk without getting short of breath.

I've seen the dialysis treatments. I've seen the large needles that are put in mom's little arms. I know she is uncomfortable sitting for three to four hours. Dialysis is difficult. But not just for the patient, it's hard for us family members too!

Week 14

There is no literature to support shortening treatments as the patient becomes older. In fact, most literature supports longer treatments equal better urea and other toxin clearance. As one ages, the fluid shifts can be more difficult and poorly tolerated. Often the answer to this difficulty is to lengthen treatments, so the fluid shifts are gentler.

The family of an older loved one is faced with the dilemma of quality of life versus quantity of life. It is never an easy conversation. Ideally, we have these conversations with the patient before we are facing this as a reality. These are conversations that *need* to occur no matter how difficult they are. Skipping treatments or shortening treatments in the aging dialysis patient never ends well. Poor dialysis can further lead to poorer nutrition, strength, alertness, as well as an increase the risk of falls, arrhythmias, and death.

Journaling Questions

1. *What does my mom/dad envision as her/his last days?*
2. *What are our options now that she is eighty, eighty-five, or ninety?*
3. *Who is available to help me with these difficult conversations?*

Information

- Dialysis is a choice. Discussing your options with your family, providers, and your other support systems (friends, social workers, mentors, church family, etc.) is imperative to making the right choice for you.
- Discussing your end-of-life wishes is important regardless of having CKD. Although difficult and perhaps awkward, these discussions will bring comfort to both you and your loved ones.
- Such discussions can bring dignity and beauty to death.
- If you decide to stop dialysis treatment, it is best to have your affairs in order. Things to consider are the following:
    o Your will
    o Signed advance directive (living will, durable health care power of attorney or health care proxy) complying with your state law
    o A durable power of attorney, complying with your state law, naming someone to act on your behalf on all matters other than medical (e.g., legal, financial, banking and business matters). Your power of attorney must be a *durable* one in order to stay in effect even if you become unable to make your own decisions or if you die.

○ An inventory, including the location of your bank, brokerage, and other financial accounts, stock and bond holdings, real estate and business records, medical and other insurance policies, pension plans and other legal papers.

○ Names, addresses, and telephone numbers of your attorney, accountant, family members, and other loved ones, friends, and business associates who should be notified of your death or who may have information that will be helpful in dealing with estate affairs.

○ A statement about your preference for funeral/memorial services, burial or cremation instructions and decisions about organ and tissue donation.

○ Written or video- or audiotaped message to family members and other loved ones, business associates and friends.

- There are many available resources that can help you process and make plans. Again, it is best to have these discussions with your loved ones as soon as possible rather than when you are grieving the imminent loss of a loved one or when you are too ill to make these decisions for yourself.
- The web pages www.kidney.org and www.funeralwise.com are just a few examples of the available resources.
- Another simple and useful tool is "Five Wishes," https://agingwithdignity.org/

Words of Comfort

The length of their lives is decided beforehand—the number of months they will live. You have settled it, and it can't be changed. (Job 14:5 GNT)

Today's Prayer

O God, I lay this burden down at the foot of the cross. I cannot bear this alone. I am so sad. It tortures me to see my mother suffer so. I entrust her care to you. Each time she boards the van and sits in the chair at the dialysis center, I depend on you. Bring to her, staff with great compassion, that care for her like she is their own mother. Comfort me as I bear this burden and struggle with my own battle of guilt and helplessness. Lord God, you are the only place I can find peace in all of this. Help me to breath, to trust, to know that you have purpose in all this pain. Comfort Mom. Comfort me. Amen.

Chapter 15

This Is Expensive
How Will I Make It?

I learned from the social worker that CKD requiring dialysis is considered a permanent disability. As a permanent disability, I am eligible for financial assistance. I have Medicare. I don't understand all this language. My pharmacy keeps asking me what part D coverage I have? I don't know what this is! The surgeon's office asked about my secondary insurance. Isn't Medicare enough?

I've lived a simple and uncomplicated life. I have a small home enough for my needs. Medicare has been enough to sustain me, but now I have traveling expenses three times a week. I have all these new medications and the access procedures. I want to maintain my independence and not have to rely on my family for help!

Week 15

For the last four months, you have been the recipient of information overload. It's okay to feel like you cannot possibly take in any more information and/or keep it all straight in your mind. Your senses have been overloaded. You have received large amounts of new data to process regarding your health, important medical decisions, and a major life change. And now, there are bills coming in, and it is likely that your income has either stayed the same or taken a huge hit.

Journaling Questions

1. Who can I talk to about my financial questions?
2. What is my primary and secondary insurance? Do I have or need to have both?
3. What is Medicare part D?

Information

- Every dialysis center employs a social worker versed in financial questions.
- CKD (ESRD) is considered a permanent disability, and your social worker will help you walk through the steps to apply for this through the department of social services.
- Transportation services and discounts are available. Your social worker will facilitate the necessary paperwork with your provider and give you step-by-step instructions during the application process.
- It is in your best interest to obtain a secondary insurance if this is affordable to you.
- Part D insurance is prescription coverage and is necessary in order to obtain your medications at the best cost.
- Some individual states may have special programs that assist in paying for kidney-related medications. Ask your social worker about applying for such programs.
- Drug companies may offer coupons for specific drugs that are expensive. Your social worker, provider, or Internet searches may lead you to such offers.
- If you receive disability, the amount of income you can earn is limited. It is very important not to supersede this amount and endanger your social security benefits. If this happens, there is a steep penalty to pay.
- Resources that you may find helpful are:
    - www.niddk.nih.gov/health-information/ kidney-disease/kidney-failure/financial
    - www.kidneyfund.org
    - www.kidney.org

Words of Comfort

Hear me, Lord, and answer me, for I am
poor and needy. (Psalm 86:1 NIV)

Today's Prayer

O Lord, hear my plea, for I am feeling needy and poor. Cast out all my anxieties about my insufficient income and heavy expenses. Cast out my worries about making ends meet when I see the bills mounting up. Lord, you are the great provider and will make a way when there seems to be no way. Increase my faithfulness. Amen.

Chapter 16

Trusting You Can Be So Hard

I want to believe that you are infallible. My very life depends on your actions and knowledge. I recognize that we all make mistakes; it is human nature. But your mistakes can cost us, your patients, dearly!

I am tired when I sit here for four hours day after day. I try to stay alert and be aware of all the activity happening to me and those I've come to consider my dialysis family. Some days I feel under par, and I just must close my eyes. I want to trust that I will be safe under your care when I let down my guard and allow myself to rest.

Certainly, you understand my reaction of fear and anger when things go wrong under your watchful eyes. Certainly, you understand that I am so grateful for you too.

Week 16

Dialysis treatments can cause you to feel sleepy especially if you are on shift one or perhaps have had a full day of appointments or other activities prior to coming. Resting and napping during treatments is perfectly natural and acceptable.

Each staff member typically cares for three people during each shift. Additionally, there is a registered nurse who assesses you, administers medications, and monitors your dialysis.

You are under careful monitoring and watchful eyes. Still unforeseen changes can occur resulting in dropped blood pressures, clotted accesses, and seizures to name a few. Rules that the staff enforce but may seem annoying to you are all in place to provide you with the safest care possible.

Journaling Questions

1. *What are the potential dangers to dialysis treatments?*
2. *What safeguards are in place to prevent these potential problems?*
3. *Are the staff prepared to handle emergencies?*

Information

- Each staff member has a three-to-one ratio, patient to staff.
- RNs are responsible for leading the team, patient management, administering of medications, physical assessments, and making any necessary adjustments to your care as deemed necessary.
- Your access site, regardless of location, must always be visible. This enables the staff to monitor for needle dislodgement and bleeding.
- Your face must be uncovered. This enables the staff to monitor for any changes in your level of consciousness
- Your rate of fluid removal must be set according to your provider's orders. Taking excessive fluids in a short period of time increases the risk for drops in blood pressure and fainting.
- All staff are trained in common emergencies such as bleeding, dropped blood pressure, dropped blood sugar, shortness of breath, cramping, infiltration of needles, etc.
- All staff are CPR certified.
- Eating/drinking during dialysis is dangerous and, therefore, limited to one small sandwich bag-sized snack.
- Because blood pressure can drop quickly and change ones mental alertness, eating large amounts can increase the risk of choking, aspiration, and death.

- Needle removal and holding of sites is done according to policy to prevent excessive/uncontrollable bleeding.
- Your blood pressure cuff should always be on bare skin and on since changes in blood pressure is a common occurrence and can result in sudden changes in your wellbeing.
- Sleeping during treatments is acceptable and safe. Your vital signs are assessed every thirty minutes to monitor for changes.

Words of Comfort

When I am afraid, I put my trust in you.
(Psalm 56:3 NIV)

Today's Prayer

Lord, you know my fears, my doubts, and my worries. You see me now and watch over me. You are always my protector. Lord, give me comfort. Allay all my fears with whom my care is entrusted. Help me to find peace during each treatment and confidence in my technicians and nurses. When troubles occur, let me shed grace to those who respond to my needs. Let me consider it pure joy when I respond to any necessary treatments and my wellbeing is restored. Amen.

Chapter 17

The Weariness of Waiting

I have been on dialysis for three years. I come to all my treatments and have been trying to wait patiently for a transplant. I became active on the list before I even started hemodialysis, and I thought I would have one by now. I've watched many friends at the clinic receive their transplants. Sometimes I feel discouraged. I'm happy for them but can't help wonder, "What about me?"

I sometimes consider stopping dialysis. What's the point? I'm never going to get one. I know this isn't logical thinking, but it's my reality. I'm sick and tired of dialysis week after week. When I mention my doubts to my providers, they try to be encouraging. They tell me how well I am doing—but I'm not! I feel like I'm living a slow death. Or they will make suggestions about discussing my transplant needs with family and friends because a live donor is quicker. I've already exhausted these avenues! My very caring providers cannot fix my problem.

So I clam up about how I am feeling. I figure there is no point in making everyone else miserable. I decide to hold these thoughts inside. I do things that aren't in my best interest. I skip Saturday treatments more frequently. I've gained weight, even though I know this jeopardizes my transplant status. Eating is the one single pleasure I still enjoy. I don't seem to have much energy to do anything else that I once enjoyed.

Week 17

There is no cure for end-stage renal disease. Your reality is to continue with some form of renal replacement therapy for the remainder of your life or to receive a kidney transplant. The process of becoming active on the transplant list for a deceased donor kidney is tedious and arduous. Weariness does not even begin to describe the waiting process. It is not uncommon to have moments in which you become discouraged and feel defeated.

Journaling Questions

1. *What emotion(s) do I experience when I hear the good news of someone else's transplant success?*
2. *What are my temptations of self-defeat when I am discouraged or weary? How can I overcome these temptations?*

Information

- The wait time for a deceased donor transplant is approximately five years.
- A deceased donor is someone who dies, is listed as an organ transplant on their driver's license, or living will and has a viable organ after death suitable for transplantation.
- Most deceased organ donations occur after tragic deaths such as vehicle accidents or irreparable brain injury to the donor.
- To be active on the transplant list, a person must be evaluated by the transplant team and meet specific criteria to ensure that organ transplantation is in the best interest of the candidate from a physical, social, and emotional perspective.
- Once active on the transplant list, it requires waiting until a suitable deceased donor organ becomes available.
- You will be responsible for making sure you have up to date diagnostics and tissue sampling while on the active list. This is communicated via your transplant coordinator, separate from your dialysis team.
- Certain characteristics increase the likelihood of earlier transplantation. These include previous transplant, years on dialysis, comorbidities, etc.

- Hepatitis C and HIV may increase the pool of donors for individuals who have these diseases.
- One stumbling block to transplant can be a high body mass index (BMI). The actual transplantation surgery is more complicated with an obese abdomen. Most transplant centers will deny candidacy for those with a BMI>40. Fortunately, your dietician can provide you with your BMI score and assist you with individualized diet plans and alternatives to reach your ideal score.
- Antihuman leukocyte antigen donor specific antibodies (anti-HLA DSAs) are measured prior to transplantation. Having a high number of different antibodies toward different tissue types can be another stumbling block for transplant.
- Anti-HLA antibodies are formed by the immune system when you are exposed to proteins that appear like tissue types. Common exposures include previous transplantation, pregnancy, or blood transfusion. Sometimes the exposure source is unknown.
- After your antibodies are measured, your transplant team can use them to calculate your *calculated panel reactive antibody or cPRA*. The cPRA gives you an idea of the percentage of offered kidneys your body would likely reject at the time of transplantation. It is harder to find compatible donor organs for those with high cPRA levels.
- Because there are many patients with antibodies against their donor, pools of incompatible donors and recipients have been formed. Paired donation with a living donor is a specialized program and matching system developed to take donors and recipients from these pools in order to create compatible matches.
- Occasionally, it is possible to undergo transplantation if you have antibodies toward your donor. This may be done at a specialized transplant center. You may need special treatments such as plasmapheresis and/or intravenous immunoglobulin (IVIG) to undergo this type of transplant. These

are treatments that can remove antibodies. In select situations, positive crossmatch kidney transplantation is a better option than remaining on the deceased donor waiting list.

- There are many altruistic individuals who are willing to donate a kidney to a nonrelated person in need. There are many ways to make your need known. Social media has become a prevalent avenue for getting the word out to many.
- Speaking to other dialysis patients may give you creative ideas, as well as encouragement, during the wait.
- Transplant is not the answer for all dialysis patients. This decision is very individualized, and there is no right/wrong answer.
- If you are uncertain that transplant is the course for you, even if you have been deemed an excellent candidate, talk to your social worker, and she/he will arrange for you to meet with former patients who have been transplanted and can give you an account of their personal experience.

Words of Comfort

> Ah, Sovereign Lord, you have made the heavens and the earth by your great power and outstretched arm. Nothing is too hard for you. (Jeremiah 32:17 NIV)

Today's Prayer

All-knowing Lord, I want to rely on your plans for me, even if they do not include a transplant tomorrow, next week, or ever. You know the desires of my heart. Help me to place my faith in your timing and not of my own. Carry me on the days when the taste of disappointment is bitter on my lips, and my temptations are too hard to bear up against. Amen.

Chapter 18

Who Makes the Rules?

I consider myself a rule-follower and rarely have I gone against the grain throughout my life. But that was before I lost complete control of as much as I have with CKD. Now I find myself forced to come to dialysis three times a week and am continually being told what I can and cannot do! No eating on the machine, no shortening my treatment, no covering my face during treatment, no bending my arm, and the list seems to go on and on. Who makes these rules and why?

Week 18

There are many *rules* to dialysis. These policies have been created to ensure safe care for you during your treatments. The staff are expected to enforce them in order to prevent injury and harm, not to be dictatorial or to usurp your voice. All these mandated rules do come with explanations, but perhaps in all the details the staff are managing, the explanations are glossed over. It is important to ask for clarification. Understanding the rules will help you to appreciate their importance and perhaps change some rules that have become dated and obsolete.

Journaling Questions

1. *Sometimes I ask questions about a rule, but I get different answers depending on who I ask. Where is the best source of information for my questions?*

2. *If I disagree or do not wish to comply with a certain rule, what is my best course of action?*

Information

- The staff at your dialysis facility are following well-established guidelines not only for your own safety and survival but also for the welfare of your dialysis unit.
- All dialysis units have a standard for issuing complaints, and it was likely in the *packet* of forms you received and signed on your very first day of dialysis. Please ask the administrative assistant to direct you with any concerns you have within your facility
- The state board also has a customer service department should you feel your concerns are not being addressed appropriately. Your social worker will be able to provide you with this contact information.
- Additionally, some dialysis centers have appointed spokespersons to address patient concerns with the medical director and healthcare team on a regular basis. If your unit does not have this system in place, perhaps you can suggest it.
- Many restrictions that patients complain about during dialysis are due to safe practices such as:
    - Covering your face or access during treatment will impede the staff's ability to assess for change in mental status, choking, fainting, and breathing difficulty and bleeding.
    - Eating large quantities of food during treatment can cause your blood pressure to decline and fainting to occur

- Excessive movement of your body/limbs during dialysis can cause dislodgement of the needles and unnecessary bleeding risks.
- Missing treatments, shortening treatments, and altering treatments need to be discussed with your provider. Failure

to do so without this discussion is like stopping medications without talking with your provider. Your treatment is individualized with your best interest in mind.

- The National Kidney Foundation produces clinical practice guidelines through the NKF Kidney Disease Outcomes Quality Initiative (NKF KDOQI).
- This program has provided evidence-based guidelines for all stages of chronic kidney disease (CKD) and related complications since 1997.
- Recognized throughout the world for improving the diagnosis and treatment of kidney disease, the KDOQI guidelines have changed the practices of numerous specialties and disciplines and improved the lives of thousands of kidney patients.
- All KDOQI Guidelines and Commentaries are published in the *American Journal of Kidney Diseases* (*AJKD*), NKF's premier journal.
- The Centers for Medicare & Medicaid Services (CMS) is part of the US Department of Health and Human Services. CMS oversees many federal healthcare programs
- The Survey and Certification Program certifies ESRD facilities for inclusion in the Medicare program by validating that the care and services of each facility meet specified safety and quality standards called "Conditions for Coverage." The Survey and Certification Program provides initial certification of each dialysis facility and ongoing monitoring to ensure that these facilities continue to meet these basic requirements.
- Failure to meet and maintain these standards identified by CMS jeopardize the accreditation of the facility and associated reimbursement by Medicare/Medicaid for services provided.
- These regulations are available at https://www.cms.gov/Center/Special-Topic/End-Stage-Renal-Disease-ESRD-Center.html

Words of Comfort

Have confidence in your leaders and submit to their authority, because they keep watch over you as those who must give an account. (Hebrews 13:17 NIV)

Today's Prayer

You are my God, ruler of everything. Help me to recognize the rules and restrictions I feel during my dialysis treatments are for my own safety. Take away any and all lies that make me feel and think otherwise. I pray for the authorities of those managing dialysis units and the integrity of every care giver. Amen.

Chapter 19

No One Listens to Me

I feel like I have no say in how I want to be treated at dialysis. If I were a child, yesterday's experience would have been called a meltdown, but because I'm a grown man, my behavior was called inappropriate and potential grounds for dismissal.

I wanted my Band-Aids reinforced. I told the tech forcefully that's what I want! I used curse words. She refused stating it was against policy, and that it could clot off my access.

The technician didn't know that after my last dialysis, I began bleeding. She didn't know that my neighbors cowered away from me as my blood spilled all over my apartment building elevator. She didn't know how embarrassed and scared I was.

The dialysis unit has rules. Rules to protect the patient, not harm them. Tight bandages can cause the access to clot off, causing a great deal of problems. I would then need to go to an access center for a declot, if that were even possible. I could lose my access altogether and end up with a catheter again.

I didn't want to listen to her explanation. I didn't tell her why I wanted a reinforced bandage. I just wanted her to do it as I asked. I wanted control. It's hard to have to ask permission on how you want your body cared for.

It makes me angry. This whole situation makes me angry, and now I'm feeling humiliated.

Week 19

You are in a very vulnerable situation. You require life-saving dialysis three times a week. You rely on the expertise and the compassion of the staff. They are competent and good at what they do. You will gain the most benefit from the dialysis team by

- realizing you are your own best advocate.
- If you do not speak up about issues you are experiencing, the staff won't be able to advise and help you.
- Sometimes you will need to listen to and hear the explanations you are being given.
- At all times, a dialogue is appropriate.
- The team wants to give you control of your care, at the same time, safety cannot be compromised.

Journaling Questions

1. *What can I control regarding my dialysis experience? And who do I ask?*
2. *What is the process for expressing concerns I might have?*

Information

- Tight bandages around the access for prolonged periods can disrupt blood flow to your fistula or graft which can cause the access to clot.
- Tight clothing, watches, or laying on the access can cause clotting.
- A clotted access is considered an urgent matter. Blood flow must be restored in a timely fashion, or the access will no longer function.
- Interventional radiology centers that specialize in dialysis accesses are readily available and are geared to accommodate dialysis patients quickly.

- A procedure can be performed that will remove the clot and restore blood flow. This is sometimes referred to as a balloon; the correct name is a percutaneous angioplasty (PTA). The access can be used immediately after the procedure.
- If too much time has lapsed, the blood flow may not be able to be restored. In such cases, a catheter will be inserted so that dialysis can be resumed.
- Bleeding from your access can occur at any time. Apply direct pressure to the site. Most of the time, this is enough. If bleeding continues call 911. *Always* report it to the staff. This may indicate a narrowing in your fistula or graft that needs an intervention.
- Any time that you notice you are having prolonged bleeding after the needles are removed, generally greater than ten to fifteen minutes, your provider needs to be notified. The staff will keep your provider aware of any bleeding concerns.
- Prolonged bleeding can be due to multiple reasons but should never be ignored.
- Common reasons for prolonged bleeding include:
  - Narrowing or occlusion of your access above the site, this may be referred to as a stenosis.
  - Too much blood thinner during treatment. The medication is called heparin; it is short acting about six hours. Some patients require none, some require a dose at the start of treatment, and some require an initial startup dose and then smaller amounts each hour while dialyzing.
  - Overuse of an area of your access, this can be prevented by rotation of the needle sites. Rotation is standard procedure, but sometimes patients request a certain area to be used over and over because there is less pain when the skin has thinned from frequent use.

- Blood makes people nervous. It is fear of the unknown. Believe it or not, you will become an expert on dealing with blood. Remember to remain calm and apply pressure.
- Anger and fear are closely connected. Your dialysis team understands this, but continual threatening behavior and foul language are not permitted. You likely signed an agreement about this when you started at the dialysis center. A behavioral contract will be initiated at the discretion of the Administrator.

Words of Comfort

> Let us then approach God's throne of grace with confidence, so that we may receive mercy and find grace to help us in our time of need. (Hebrews 4:16 NIV)

Today's Prayer

Lord, I beseech you to help the staff to remember how difficult this is for us who sit in these chairs. Please reassure the staff that we appreciate their skill and knowledge. Give them sufficient forgiveness and compassion for when I act out of character. Help the staff hear me, even when I am not clear with my choice of words. Lord, help me to be a better listener. Amen.

Chapter 20

One Day at a Time

This first year has not been easy. I was told to expect to feel better, and I was counting on it. Unfortunately for me, it seems like it has been one blow after another. My kidneys failed; now I have been told I have kidney cancer. This means I can't even start to think about a transplant until after surgery and waiting two years. And that's the best-case scenario. I feel hopeless, at least when it comes to my health and my future.

I've always considered myself a man of faith. My faith has been challenged like never before. I feel like my entire life is crumbling. My health, my relationships, and my faith, all feel wobbly. The best I can do is take one day at a time.

Week 20

Many times, kidney disease is discovered in the setting of many other health conditions. This often results in figuring out your health priorities as you are being given more and more bad news about what isn't working in your body! Your best decisions can only be made with the information you are being given and the resources you have available. We all know what the "ivory tower" of life is supposed to be, but few live this reality.

Taking it one day at a time is not bad advice. In doing so, you are forced to live in the here and now and not worry about the future. No health care provider, friend, loved one, or you know what lies ahead. Therefore, dealing with today's issue and the information you have in this moment is *all* that you can use to make this the best day it can be.

Journaling Questions

1. *What is my biggest challenge today? This week? This month?*
2. *What answers do I need to help me make the best choices for facing this challenge?*

Information

- Kidney health not only depends on the function of other organs, but kidney disease also affects the function of your blood cell production, bone health, and heart.
- The top causes of kidney disease are diabetes and hypertension. These diseases still need to be controlled despite the permanent damage that has already happened to your kidneys.
- Failure to maintain glucose control can further weaken your immune system and cause progressive vascular disease, nerve damage, and affects your heart and eye health to name a few.
- If you have diabetes, it is in your best interest to be followed by the diabetic or endocrine clinic. Most of these clinics give comprehensive care including podiatry, ophthalmology, and dietary counsel.
- Hypertension or high blood pressure is often managed by your nephrology team at the dialysis center; however, involvement with your PCP is in your best interest to monitor for other associated complications such as cardiac health and ophthalmology care.
- Many other conditions may have precipitated your kidney disease. Examples are autoimmune diseases like Lupus, congenital defects, inheritable diseases such as sickle cell or polycystic disease. Whatever the cause or your disease, it is important to continue receiving routine follow-up for these conditions as the nephrology team is limited in time and ability to follow other conditions thoroughly.
- Renal cell cancer (RCC) or kidney cancer can occur as the primary cause of your kidney failure or can occur even

years after you have been receiving dialysis. RCC is curative with a nephrectomy or surgical removal of the kidney. Your provider may order routine CT scans to follow any kidney masses/cysts that you currently have.

- Kidney disease is a *chronic* health condition. It is not curable. Therefore, approaching the diagnosis as a part of your life may give you a healthy outlook to developing coping skills to the associated ups and downs that come with any *chronic* illness.
- A healthy outlook does not come in the form of an easy formula. At the very minimum, it entails enlisting a strong support system, a trusting and mutual listening rapport with your healthcare team. A faith-based lifestyle has shown to offer comfort and peace to many.
- Exploring your fears, unlived dreams, and expectations of your remaining years is a good way to begin. Specific formal resources are difficult to find but are available.

Words of Comfort

Have mercy on me, Lord, for I am faint; heal me, Lord, for my bones are in agony. My soul is in deep anguish. How long, Lord, how long? Turn, Lord, and deliver me; save me because of your unfailing love. Among the dead no one proclaims your name. Who praises you from the grave? I am worn out from groaning. All night long I flood my bed with weeping and drench my couch with tears. My eyes grow weak with sorrow; they fail because of all my foes. Away from me, all you who do evil, for the Lord has heard my weeping. (Psalm 6:2–8 NIV)

Today's Prayer

Creator, you know me better than I know myself. You know my worries that I cannot even put into words. You are my only hope. That's hard to admit. I am so used to taking control of things, but in this disease, I feel powerless. I submit my every ache, my every pain, and my every need to you. Comfort me now and with each new challenge that presents itself. I trust that you hear my weeping and will dry my tears with the hope that only you can bring. Amen.

Chapter 21

Not Today

*Unless you have walked a day in my life, you can't really under-
stand how monotonous this becomes. I'm told that my life depends on
my coming to each treatment no matter what! I'm told that dialysis takes
priority over everything!*

*To my team and to this sentiment, I say, "You try it." Look, I realize
how important HD is. I realize if I miss a treatment, I jeopardize my
breathing, my interdialytic weight gain will be high, and I even risk my
life due to a sudden irregular heartbeat related to a high potassium.*

*It's not as though I want to play "Russian roulette" with my life.
I want to take care of myself. Sometimes it feels like the providers don't
understand. I have responsibilities just like you. My car sometimes breaks
down, just like yours. My kids get sick, just like yours do. I have off days,
just like you do.*

Week 21

Employers give staff time off. Some companies make this man-
datory, recognizing that work performance is enhanced by having
vacation days to regroup and refuel. Unfortunately, when it comes
to dialysis, there is no safe way to "take time off." It is different than
most other life experiences.

Changing your mindset about dialysis from being *something you
must do* to a perspective of *I'm able to do* will help tremendously with
your motivation. When we feel we are obligated to do something
we don't particularly like, the activity can become one we dread and

bemoan. Thinking of dialysis as a healthy step toward your well-being makes it an activity that we feel privileged by and glad for.

You may think this is just a play on words or a way of deluding yourself. Maybe. But the sooner you develop coping skills, the sooner you will adjust to having dialysis be a part of your life like any other necessary activity.

Many equate HD to a work schedule, but as mentioned above, with work, you get days off. With HD, there isn't a built-in vacation. Hemodialysis is a life-sustaining necessity for you.

Ideas such as making a lunch date once a week, planning a long weekend by altering you HD schedule once a quarter, or even traveling to another location and doing HD in a visiting unit can bring an improved attitude toward the monotony.

Options are available other than in center HD such has home HD and PD. These also require dedication, compliance, and perseverance in order to be successful.

Journaling Questions

1. What is it that makes me dread HD the most?
2. Is there any way to change this?
3. What am I supposed to do when something else of equal importance falls on a scheduled dialysis day?

Information

- Adequacy of dialysis is measured monthly by blood work. This is often referred to as urea clearance or KT/V.
- KT/V is a calculation derived at by the dialyzers clearance of urea (K) multiplied by the duration of the dialysis treatment (t in minutes) divided by the volume of distribution of urea in the body (V in mL). In short, it is a complex equation used to determine the removal of known toxins based on your dialysis prescription and body surface area.
- The KDOQI guidelines recommend achieving a KT/V of 1.2 as the minimal number necessary for adequate dialysis.

- When the KT/V is below 1.2, it may indicate that longer treatment times are necessary or a larger dialyzer is required, or it may indicate that there is an issue with your access.
- Many dialysis centers also obtain monthly flow studies. These studies when combined with other findings can be helpful in detecting access issues such as a narrowing.
- The standard for in-center dialysis is three times weekly. Some alterations can be made in schedules such as days of the week, but anything less than thrice weekly treatment is considered inadequate nationally.
- Vacationing is permissible but only when obtaining dialysis during the vacation following a similar schedule/prescription as your standard one.
- When planning a vacation, your social worker or administrative assistant will need specifics from you such as dates of travel, address of your vacation spot, and up-to-date insurance information. With this data, a dialysis center will be located near your vacation spot, and a request is placed for an available spot for you to be dialyzed.
- Transportation to and from the "transient center" is your responsibility.
- Once the details above are finalized, your HD center will send all necessary paperwork. This typically includes insurance verification, a recent history and physical from your doctor, updated labs specifically PPD and hepatitis B information. Also, a copy of your current HD prescription will be sent to the transient center.
- The providers at the transient center write the orders for your visit. Sometimes, the dialyzer may differ, or your in-center medications may not be available. Be assured that these are minor differences and should not be a deterrent for vacationing.
- Home hemodialysis (HHD) is an alternative to in-center HD and is becoming more and more prevalent. The emphasis for HHD is partially due to the financial burden of in-center HD on Medicare/Medicaid but also in hopes for greater patient satisfaction and compliance.

- HHD allows you to receive a similar type of HD, but you are in charge of your treatments; therefore, it gives you much greater flexibility, eliminates the transportation time, and has equal outcomes to in-center.
- Peritoneal HD is an alternative type of dialysis that achieves the same outcomes.
- PD requires a catheter to be placed in your left lower abdomen that is permanent. This is performed as an outpatient and is done by an interventional radiologist.
- The PD catheter is a free-floating catheter that uses your own peritoneum (lining between your intestines and abdominal wall) as the dialyzer.
- Both PD and HHD have extensive one on one training classes for you and your family. You also will have easy and quick access to staff for problem solving any issues.
- When choosing an in-center dialysis unit, ask specific questions about schedule flexibility. What are the policies for requesting different shifts or schedules? How accommodating is the unit to patient needs?
- Schedules do have constraints in busy dialysis units; however, these centers do monitor missed treatments and, therefore, are interested in making sure you do not miss yours. Be assured they will work with you when life happens.

Words of Comfort

Come to me, all you who are weary and burdened, and I will give you rest." For my yoke is easy and burden light. (Matthew 11:28, 30 NIV)

Today's Prayer

Lord, only you know the true burden I carry. Dialysis is just one piece of my life. Sometimes it feels like no one understands this. I know the team of professionals are giving me information to improve my chances of survival. I know coming to dialysis is good and right. But you know how hard this is for me. Lord, I invite you to help carry my load, for without you, I cannot continue. Lord God, may your strength carry me today. Amen.

Chapter 22

Substance and Sustenance

Life on hemodialysis can be restrictive, stifling, and full of pain. Regardless of the cause of your CKD, once you receive the diagnosis, there is no going back. I developed CKD from HIV resulting from drug use. In the beginning—and to be honest, on occasion even now—I cover up my pain (physical and emotional) with drugs, an extra oxycodone, a fifth of vodka, a hit of crack, or a snort of heroin.

If you've never used or abused drugs, I get why you want to stop reading this and dismiss me for getting what I deserve. I understand. But if you are so inclined, please keep reading. Our journey is the same, but we've chosen different paths.

I realize now that I didn't learn/choose healthy coping mechanisms. Mine was a path of survival. Doing what I knew to get by, get through, and get on. Using substances for other than their intended or prescribed use is drug abuse—that is the definition.

So if I know this, and I know I'm further harming myself, why do I sometimes abuse? Risking judgement and other unforeseen potential losses, including my very life? That is the million-dollar question. Why do I do the things I don't want to instead of doing the things I do want to do? All people, abusers or not, Christian or not, with good kidney function or not, have asked themselves this.

It is human nature, choice, free will, or whatever you prefer to call it. It's easier to see someone else's fault/sin and condemn than our very own. Please try to remember this when I come in stoned or don't show up at all. Love me and judge me as you would have others love and judge you.

Week 22

Usually by this point in your dialysis treatment, some of the old patterns can return. It's easier to pay attention to rules and do what is best for yourself when you are still feeling poorly and see that the treatments improve your health. As time goes on, the monotony can set in, and the commitment to your own health can dwindle. Missing treatments and engaging in poor choices, addictions, and unhealthy behaviors can resurface. Usually it is not *if*, it is *when* they resurface.

It may feel as though you receive judgement from the clinic staff and your fellow comrades when these behaviors are addressed. With all addictions, there comes self-condemnation as well.

Addressing these habits sooner rather than later are very important in developing an action plan. Pretending that they do not exist or are not noticeable is a farce. There are resources and mechanisms to tap into for learning healthier coping strategies. Do not be afraid to acknowledge that you will need help.

Journaling Questions

1. *What are one to two healthy choices I can make when temptations seize me?*
2. *What are my triggers that produce the "perfect storm" within me?*

Information

- Many things can cause CKD. The two most prevalent are diabetes and uncontrolled hypertension.
- Alcohol and drug abuse place an individual at higher risk for kidney disease.
- Coma due to overdose can lead to rhabdomyolysis, a condition characterized by the breakdown of muscle tissue and release of proteins into the blood. One of these proteins is myoglobin, which can cause obstruction and kidney damage. Dehydration, acidosis, low blood pressure, and oxygen deficiency can exacerbate these effects.

- Rhabdomyolysis is commonly seen in those who abuse cocaine, and some go on to develop acute kidney failure.
- Cocaine abuse can lead to *renal infarction*, as well as promote atherosclerosis, or plaque buildup in the renal arterial walls—conditions that are both characterized by disruptions in blood flow to the kidney and result in tissue damage.
- Acute renal failure or injury may be caused by malignant hypertension or severely high blood pressure, which can result from or be exacerbated by MDMA use.
- Alcohol can directly affect the kidney through binge drinking or through repetitive drinking. Drinking alcohol can change/damage the structure and function of the kidney leading to chronic problems.
- Most drugs such as heroin, cocaine, MDMA, and alcohol are dialyzed out of the system. Therefore, if you abuse substance while being dialyzed, you can go through acute withdraw.

Words of Comfort

Watch and pray so that you will not fall into temptation. The spirit is willing, but the flesh is weak. (Matthew 26:41 NIV)

Today's Prayer

Forgive me, Father, for my weak flesh. Forgive me, Father, for those moments when I quiver with desire for those things which cause me more harm. O Lord, stop this battle within me and help me to recognize the temptations and to lean on you each time they are triggered within me. Lord God, help those caring for me to extend grace and love when I fall. Help them to appreciate how I long to stop this cycle of shame and to be healed.

Chapter 23

And Now They Are Gone

It would be difficult to work in a chronic hemodialysis unit and not get attached to those we care for...even those that are grumpy! We spend a great deal of time together every week. It may not seem like an abundance of time, ten minutes here, ten minutes there, but all these moments add up to bring meaningful relationship to all our lives.

I mourn your losses. Albeit differently than you, but with every setback, every access loss, every health challenge, I empathize. A concept rarely spoken of between patient and health care worker, we are doing life together. The HD unit is unique in this way. I've known some of my patients longer then my spouse. I've listened to your story, and you've listened to mine. We are woven into each other's story. I recognize and consider this a huge privilege.

Week 23

The outpatient hemodialysis unit is both static and dynamic. Dynamic in that it can seem like a revolving door with new patients and staff coming and going every day. This is true for a variety of reasons. Patients may be assigned to your unit temporarily until a spot closer to their home opens. This is reasonable. Some patients present to HD at the end of their lives and, therefore, have a short-sustained time at the unit. Similar reasons exist for staff.

The unit is also static in nature, meaning there are many long-term patients and staff. It is in this setting where relationships grow beyond the typical patient/care provider relationship. Anytime one has relationship for an extended period, greater fondness and familiarity develop. There is great comfort in knowing and being known by someone, and this is one of the blessings of the HD unit. Memories live on long beyond the time spent together. It is in these memories that you realize how rich your lives are because of the day-to-day moments.

Journaling Questions

1. *What part of my story do I want others to know?*
2. *Is there greater purpose in the connection of our lives?*

Information

- The average survival rate, according to statistics, is five years after being diagnosed with CKD stage 5, but many have lived on dialysis ten to twenty years.
- According to US Renal Data System, the mortality rate is twice as high for dialysis patients aged sixty-five and above in comparison to the general population who have diabetes, cancer, congestive heart failure, CVA/TIA, or AMI.
- The five-year survival rates after the start of dialysis for diabetes, polycystic kidney disease, and glomerulonephritis are about 29 percent, 70 percent, and 58 percent respectively.
- The dialysis unit, the other patients, and the staff will all become part of your life. This is not by choice but rather circumstance. Because of this fact, it is not unusual to develop feelings like that of a family.
- As in traditional families, the dialysis family may experience joy, celebration, sadness, and resentment, days where you lash out and days where you love them to pieces.
- "Grumpy" days happen with and without CKD. The staff are trained to assess for other causes if there is a notable change in behavior. Uremia or the buildup of waste products in the blood can produce out of character behavior.

Medications and infection can also alter one's mental status and coping mechanisms.

- Secure attachment does occur between patient and staff and patient to patient in the dialysis environment. This type of attachment takes place when there is trust, dependence, honest communication, and forgiveness.
- It is not unusual or abnormal to mourn each other's losses or be filled with joy in one another's celebrations.
- Dialysis centers have full-time licensed social workers who are available to help with your adjustment to CKD, losses, etc.
- Professional counselors or lay counselors may be helpful as well.
- Some believe in coincidences; some believe in divine intervention. Regardless, our lives are interwoven and connected. It is up to each of us as individuals to determine the outcome of these interactions.

Words of Comfort

Rejoice with those who rejoice; mourn with those who mourn. (Romans 12:15 NIV)

Today's Prayer

Lord, I don't know why you brought me to this place and this time with these people? I don't know if I am faithful enough to consider it all part of your divine plan? I do know that you are present in my life in all circumstances. Help me to embrace and love without reserve those present in my life today. Amen.

Chapter 24

No Condemnation

As a provider of care to those of you with chronic kidney disease, I am intrigued each time I meet a new patient. Intrigued by your story, your coping process, and your challenges. Although the disease and the treatment carry great similarities among my patients, rarely is the journey ever the same.

I have learned many things about this journey through each one of my patients. Probably one of the most important that I would like to share is that there is no place for condemnation. Living with dialysis is a hard road. It is one that causes understandable denial. It can take some soul-searching and hard work to uncover your personal sources of this resistance. For some, the denial lasts much longer than others and often surfaces in unhealthy choices.

Like myself, your care provider wants to know upfront and foremost what your goals are. In the beginning, common goals are to feel better, regain my strength, and to live! As months go by, years go by, and decades go by, these goals change. Your provider can quote the latest research findings on the best approach to your care, and although this is extremely important, it may not be your priority in this juncture of your journey.

As a provider, it is our goal to assist you in the quality of life you desire within the constraints of life-sustaining hemodialysis three times per week. Open dialogue is key to assuring you of the highest quality possible.

Disagreement does not equal condemnation. Communicating your goals is of utmost importance to living a quality life with CKD.

Week 24

You have been receiving dialysis treatments for approximately six months at this point. A great deal of this time has been focused on your health. Fitting hemodialysis treatments three times per week into your life has not been easy. You may have skipped days, shortened treatments, or been hospitalized.

You may have missed important events in your life including family milestones, holidays, and vacations.

You may have even had the experience of defeat and failure. You have tried to follow the recommendations of your physician and care team and despite your best efforts…there have been setbacks, disappointments, and suboptimal progress.

Journaling Questions

1. *How can I still do all the things I desire and still do what I am supposed to do for my health?*
2. *What advice is there on handling those times in my life when a priority is greater to me than my dialysis treatment?*

Information

- The standard of care for hemodialysis in the USA is attending thrice weekly sessions. For most centers, this means following a Monday/Wednesday/Friday schedule or a Tuesday/Thursday/Saturday schedule.
- The prescription of duration of your dialysis sessions is determined by your nephrologist and based on the adequacy of urea reduction, a monthly lab test.
- Other determinants factored into the duration of your treatment time is your ability to manage fluids and fluid removal.
- Dialysis via an arteriovenous fistula (AVF) or arteriovenous graft (AVG) is recommended. Catheters are only suitable for those with medical conditions that prohibit an AVF/AVG from being placed.

- Other dialysis modalities are available such as peritoneal dialysis (PD) and home hemodialysis (HH) and can be discussed with your team at any time.
- Exclusions from PD include extensive abdominal surgery history, abdominal hernias, poorly controlled DM, or lack of resources/social support.
- Exclusions from HH include lack of social support systems, having a catheter, and inability to self-cannulate.
- Some areas offer a nighttime hemodialysis unit to accommodate those working during the day hours.
- Most dialysis units offer flexibility with a requested schedule change, but you must preplan schedule changes.
- Communicating with your provider and dialysis center team is in your own best interest. Your providers empathize with your restrictions, and although they cannot fix every situation, they are eager to work with you to make the best decision in every given scenario.
- Schedule changes and life's demands require out-of-the-box thinking at times. An open dialogue is the *only* way to get the best advice for such times.
- Holidays can be incredibly challenging. It will require flexibility of your family and friends in planning events and even food challenges. Involve them to help reduce your own burden and stress.
- Talking to your support system, whoever that is for you, about your struggles with CKD and life on HD will hold you accountable. Family are welcome to meet your dialysis team and discuss *any* issues you are challenged by. Most times, your social worker will coordinate such meetings.
- Not everyone is going to adhere to the advice given to them. In part, this is human nature. We make choices to the best of our ability at the given time. Unfortunately, nonadherence to dialysis, fluid restriction, and diet in the HD patient can be costly. It may result in hospitalization or even death. *Knowledge* about how best to care for yourself in these scenarios is imperative to your survival.

- For some, medications that rid the body of extra potassium is necessary.
- For some, additional treatments may become necessary.
- For some, medication delivery to the dialysis unit is helpful.
- These are just a few examples of how adjustments can be made to individualize your care based on each need.

Words of Comfort

We pray that you'll have the strength to stick it out over the long haul—not the grim strength of gritting your teeth but the glory-strength God gives. It is strength that endures the unendurable and spills over into joy. (Colossians 1:11 MSG)

Today's Prayer

Heavenly Host, through these challenges, let me not get down hearted from choosing other priorities over my health and then feeling the consequences not only physically but like a failure. Lord, these struggles, these battles I face day after day, let them build in me, perseverance so that I may resemble you in character. I am faithful that your character will prevail in me. Amen.

Chapter 25

No Begging Please!

Today is one of those days when dialysis is not going well. I feel off, and I don't want to explain it to anyone. I just need to go home.

I can't sit here another minute. I know this is not a good decision for my physical health, but for my mental health? It is just what I need to do. Your well-intentioned information, telling me what is best for me, isn't going to change my mind today. So please stop begging me to do what you want me to do, even if it is best. Please don't bargain with me to stay for another ten, fifteen, or thirty minutes. I'm not going to change my mind, and your insistence is only making me angry.

I know you are doing your job, but I am an adult, and I have ultimate control of my healthcare. Please do not lose sight of this!

Week 25

By now, you fully appreciate the consequences of shortened or missed treatment time. This does not negate the importance and emphasis placed on full treatment time. It is for obvious reasons. Shortened treatment time equals increased hospitalizations and death. The staff would be negligent if they did not try. *Bargaining* with you to accommodate your needs while providing a full treatment is the norm. Many times, it is a simple adjustment that can make all the difference. Perhaps you need a cooler environment or repositioned or headphones to drown out noise. Perhaps there is *nothing* that can convince you to stay.

Journaling Questions?

1. *How do I convince others when my no means no?*
2. *What is the truth to my skimming a few moments off my treatment time?*

Information

- One absence due to a nonmedical reason is associated with a 40 percent greater risk of hospitalization.
- Studies show that in-center dialysis patients miss about fifteen treatments per year, one-half of these missed treatments being nonmedical related.
- Absenteeism is tracked and monitored by individual dialysis units.
- A standard of care for hemodialysis patients is achieving a KT/V >1.2. KT/V is a measure of clearance of the toxin UREA.
- Urea clearance is influenced by many factors:
  - Time on dialysis
  - Size of patient (height, weight, and muscle mass)
  - Blood flow rate and dialysate flow rate
  - Size and type of dialyzer
  - Access (catheter, fistula, graft)

- Studies show that a KT/V >1.2 is associated with better survival
- Longer treatment times have been associated with the following benefits:
  - Less cramping
  - Less episodes of low blood pressure during treatment
  - Better phosphate control
  - Higher albumin levels
  - Overall better blood pressure control

○ Lower risk of sudden death and cardiovascular death (sessions of four hours)
○ Better survival

- To put it simply, missing dialysis time affects everything. This fact motivates the staff to try and convince you to complete your prescribed treatments.
- You cannot be kept on the dialysis machine against your wishes. Simply state your intent, sign the forms indicating you are shortening your treatment against medical advice, and wait patiently until your treatment is discontinued.
- When it seems impossible for you to stay for a full treatment, speak with the charge nurse to see what options are available. Perhaps an additional ultrafiltration treatment can be scheduled. Ultra filtration is a shorter period of time that removes fluid only. It does not clean the blood. It must be approved by your provider.
- If shortening your treatments becomes a pattern, your health will be affected. Therefore, if there is underlying anxiety, pain, or other reasons causing this habit, speak to your healthcare team. Developing a strategy that is less detrimental to your health may be possible when working together.
- Identifying the underlying source of anger, anxiety, or sadness is important to your coping with HD. Sometimes, we only see the tip of the iceberg to the real feelings and emotions that are deeper. Professional counsel is often necessary to help sort through these emotions. Your team can give you contact names/numbers for counseling services.

Words of Comfort

Be gentle with one another, sensitive. Forgive one another as quickly and thoroughly as God in Christ forgave you. (Ephesians 4:32 MSG)

Today's Prayer

Dear God, there are days when I'm weak. That is the truth, please understand and do not heap criticism and self-loathing on top of my bad day. O Lord, I trust that you will carry me when I am weak. Protect me when I cannot be comforted by your spirit to do the right thing. Forgive me my unloving thoughts and words to those who dare to speak into my hurt, when I cannot hear. Help those I hurt and disappoint with my words and actions. Help them to understand that my choice is not a reflection on them in any way. Amen.

Chapter 26

When the Light Dims

Today there was a hush in the unit that was palpable. The staff seemed reserved and unusually quiet. Before long, the reason was revealed. One of my fellow patients had collapsed at home and was not able to be resuscitated. Death is part of life, a celebration depending on your belief system, so not unexpected in a dialysis unit. So why was today's somber atmosphere so prominent? Because today, we lost a bright light! This individual had a presence that even in the worst of days made you feel better by his contagious smile. Despite suffering from calciphylaxis, he made others feel better through his words, his hugs, and his heart. In honor of his memory, it is fitting that the lights be dimmed today.

Week 26

Suffering and death are part of life for everyone. It is especially common in the lives of those with CKD. Despite the rules about protected health information (PHI), our dialysis units are a caring environment, much like a family. Yes, there is such a thing as the letter of the law regarding confidentiality of health information, but most importantly, there is the spirit of the law, which is love. I would rather foster a loving atmosphere where each life matters. What a comfort to know that our being made a difference, and our absence is noticeable. Shouldn't we all aim to make a significant contribution to our worlds? No matter how small, knowing our life made a difference to someone else's is the most important contribution we can hope for, and it is as simple as being kind.

Gina Novak

Journaling Questions

1. *How do I wish to be remembered?*
2. *What are some ways that I brighten the days of my dialysis unit?*
3. *Are there resources available for dealing with loss and grief?*

Information

- Cardiovascular disease (CVD) is the most common cause of death in the CKD population.
- CVD is more prevalent due to the imbalance of calcium and phosphorus in CKD.
- Great emphasis is placed on managing your bone mineral metabolism laboratory values (calcium, phosphorus, and PTH)
- Calciphylaxis is a condition that occurs with a prolonged imbalance, resulting in calcification.
- Severe calcification can result in open painful wounds of the skin.
- The treatment for calcification is pain management and administering an intravenous medication with dialysis.
- The medication is sodium thiosulfate. The exact mechanism of action is unknown, but it is thought to be a potent antioxidant and anti-inflammatory.
- Disease progression and death are realities of CKD as with any chronic condition. It is important to process your own beliefs and thoughts about death, have conversations with those closest to you, and come to an understanding about your own wishes.
- Grieving is different for everyone, but there also are commonalities. There is a large body of information on grief available to you, starting with your social worker.
- Protected health information is important, and policies must be adhered to; however, when a member of your dialysis family dies, it is equally important to discuss and process your feelings. This is true for both patients and staff.

- Many times, patients become good friends, exchange phone numbers, socialize, etc. This must be considered above legalistic rules that govern health care.

Words of Comfort

He heals the heartbroken and bandages their wounds. (Psalm 147:3 MSG)

Today's Prayer

Lord, I look to you for my help and my solace. I trust in your promise that in heaven, there will be no suffering. I long for the day when I will be reunited with you and all those who have gone before me. I look forward to a new body resurrected in you. Amen.

Chapter 27

Needles, Needles, and More Needles

As a dialysis patient, you never get completely used to the two needles placed in your arms three times a week. Some days, I barely notice them. Some days, there is a sharp pain initially that subsides quickly. Some days, a dull pinch would last for my entire treatment. It should not be surprising then that I do not react positively to the thought of more needles...influenza vaccines, hepatitis vaccines, PPD, and pneumonia vaccines! I feel like a pincushion.

Week 27

As a new patient, the hemodialysis unit requires an updated hepatitis B status, as well as proof that you do not have active tuberculosis. Once you begin dialysis, you will be requested to have annual "flu shots" and a pneumonia vaccine. These are both considered protective immunizations, as CKD is a chronic condition which makes you more susceptible to influenza and pneumonia.

Hepatitis B is a preventable blood/bodily fluid infection. Knowing your hepatitis B immunity status determines the safety of your seating among other patients and, therefore, a required blood test.

Proper education about each of the vaccines will help you to appreciate their importance and giving of your consent. Not all are *required* but strongly advised for your protection. It's important to ask questions and discuss your concerns with the staff. Education to improve your understanding is readily available.

Journaling Questions

1. *Are there any other options for dialysis that do not require needles?*
2. *What additional needles can I expect and why? How often?*

Information

- The Center for Disease Control (CDC) recommends dialysis patients and staff to be vaccinated against hepatitis B.
- Vaccination involves a series three or four injections, depending on the brand.
- The injections are given into the muscle, usually in the deltoid (upper arm) of the nonaccess arm.
- The series of injections occur over six months.
- Once vaccinated, a blood test will determine your immunity against contracting the virus.
- Occasionally the antibody level will fall below the standard, and a booster injection will be recommended.
- Hepatitis B is a viral infection spread by contact with blood or body fluids of an infected person. It is not airborne!
- Influenza or "flu shots" are offered each year and highly recommended. These are typically offered in the early fall. Although there is no guarantee to preventing acquiring the flu, it is more likely that the duration and symptoms will be much less if you do acquire the flu.
- PPD testing determines one's exposure to tuberculosis. Chest X-rays are another way to determine your exposure. This is often a required test if you are visiting another dialysis unit on vacation.
- Pneumonia vaccines are also recommended for the dialysis patient. This immunization is given once and repeated in five years.
- All immunizations should be coordinated between your dialysis unit and other providers.

- There is now an electronic system called immune-net that has been introduced to help your providers from "over-immunizing." Remember it is in your best interest to be immunized against these preventable illnesses.
- Hemodialysis requires access to one's bloodstream. Use of two needles for each treatment cannot be avoided.
- In rare instances, patients may have long-term catheters. These have a very high association with bloodstream infections, scarring of the large vessels of your neck or chest, and inadequate dialysis. If you are a long-term catheter patient, you will not be getting needles with each treatment but rather dressing changes and marked limitations to your activities of daily living.
- The *buttonhole* technique is an alternative to new needle punctures with each dialysis. This technique utilizes a track formation into your skin and then accessed, much like pierced ears. With each treatment, the patient takes an implement to remove the scabs from one's venipuncture sites and then a special made, dull rather than sharp, needle is used to pierce the skin. The needle follows the track to enter the bloodstream for dialysis. Success of the button-hole technique varies, and it waxes and wanes in popularity.

Words of Comfort

I consider that the sufferings of this present time are not worth comparing with the glory that is to be revealed to us. (Romans 8:18 NIV)

Today's Prayer

Savior, thank you for comforting me in my suffering. Remind me that I will one day be healed and perfect again. Help me to cling to your eternal promises when my hope dries up and my tolerance to today's suffering overcomes me. I place my trust in you, Lord. Amen.

Chapter 28

Alarms, Bells, and Whistles

Before starting dialysis, when I thought of medical clinics, I thought...clean, sterile environments that were eerily quiet with respect for the ill. Friends, let me tell you this is not an accurate picture of a hemodialysis unit. Not only is the environment brightly lit and chaotic at times, it also has noises that can be unbearable. It took me some time not to react to every little sound thinking that there was an emergency.

Week 28

By now, you have experienced numerous sounds in the dialysis unit. There isn't any written material provided or even a heads up from the staff that can prepare you for the noises of a working dialysis unit. In addition to the alarms set on each of the dialysis machines, there are alarms for the water system, reminder alarms for staff to perform important duties, overhead paging, and the constant drone of thirty-plus people talking.

Journaling Questions

1. *What sounds should be cause for concern?*
2. *How do I learn these important alarms? How should I respond?*

Information

- Each dialysis machine is manufactured with an alarm system to provide safe delivery of dialysis.
- Arterial pressure alarms monitor for a safe negative pressure between the arterial needle and the speed for which the machine is pulling it. If this pressure becomes increasingly negative beyond the set parameter, the blood pump stops. A staff member may need to readjust the needle position or lower the pump speed.
- Venous pressure alarms monitor the pressure in the tubing between the venous needle and blood pump. The alarm activates if the pump is pushing blood faster than your needle can receive it. Again, the blood pump stops until a staff member assesses the needle positioning or lowers the pump speed.
- The conductivity alarm monitors for proper concentrations of chemicals dissolved in the dialysate solution. If the conductivity becomes out of range, the machine will open a bypass valve and dump the dialysate down the drain.
- The temperature alarm measures the temperature of the dialysate. If the temperature becomes too high, blood cells can be damaged. If too low, you may feel cold. The bypass valve will open and dump the dialysate to keep you safe. Your provider may use temperature to help regulate blood pressure during treatment.
- The air sensor alarm monitors for excessive air in the blood tubing. If air is detected, the pump will stop, and close the venous clamp so that you cannot receive any air.
- The blood leak detector assures that blood does not leak out of the dialyzer and into the dialysate. If this happens, you will require a new dialyzer set up to prevent bacteria from entering the system.
- All technicians are board certified to understand, solve problems, and correct all systems within your machine. Additionally, the dialysis units have biomedical techni-

cians available twenty-four hours for seven days per week. Dialysis units keep extra machines readily available should there be a malfunction. This ensures that you can still receive your treatment safely and as prescribed.

- The units are well lighted for safety. A dimly lit, quiet environment is *not* a realistic expectation of the dialysis unit.
- In general, the dialysis unit can be a social environment. Most centers provide televisions for each chair, but headsets are required to keep noise to a minimum. Some listen to music; some centers may have centralized music, which contribute to the level of noise. Combined with twenty to thirty patients, ten staff members, and the conversations required to care for everyone, the noise level is always present.

Words of Comfort

But, I trust in you, Lord; you are my God.
My times are in your hands. (Psalm 31:14 NIV)

Today's Prayer

Lord, there is no greater protection than you, my rock. All other hope is sinking sand. You protect me like no other. In this, I trust. Amen.

Chapter 29

How Am I Really Doing?

I often find myself wondering when my luck will run out, and I will be at the end of the road. As I see others deteriorate week after week, it is hard to deny that this is the course of this disease. So I ask, "Will I travel a similar road? Is this the future in store for me? Is there anything I can do to avoid this path? How close am I? How am I really doing?"

Week 29

The in-center dialysis unit is a close and intimate atmosphere. Yes, every attempt is made to protect privacy, but even in the best of attempts, in-center dialysis is a shared experience. It is impossible to hide one's bad days. It's impossible to ignore the loss that occurs, loss of function and of life. These thoughts and questions are a healthy processing of the realities of CKD. Knowing what questions to ask and what *your* concerns are is an excellent starting place.

Journaling Questions

1. *What can I do to preserve and maintain my health?*
2. *What can I anticipate in the course of my disease?*

Information

- Preserving residual renal function for as long as possible is always to your benefit but not always within in your control.

- Preserving renal function means to avoid any further damage to your remaining kidney function. Although you require hemodialysis, your kidneys may have some residual function.
- Residual renal function can provide you with better volume control in the form of urine output, meaning you will not need to restrict your fluid intake as stringently.
- Residual renal function can provide your body with enough production of erythropoietin, which will help you avoid anemia associated with CKD.
- Residual renal function can provide your body with enough vitamin D production, which will help you to avoid bone disease and require less vitamin D supplementation.
- Toxins to avoid in order to preserve renal function are contrast dyes, nonsteroidal anti-inflammatory medications (Advil, Motrin, Naprosyn, Aleve), and inappropriate dosing of antibiotics.
- Adhering to your prescribed dialysis is the most important factor to preventing deterioration in your disease process.
- Skipping and shortening treatments will significantly increase your risk for a shortened life expectancy and death.
- Occasionally you will meet a HD patient who has been on dialysis for fifteen-plus years and does not always adhere to their prescribed treatment. Please *note* this is a rare exception and is *not* a proven practice but rather…luck.
- Being invested and knowledgeable about your blood work, access, and medications is another practice that will help you to avoid complications. Keep track of your individual problem areas, ask questions, and stay informed about your health.

Words of Comfort

Therefore do not worry about tomorrow, for tomorrow will worry about itself. Each day has enough trouble of its own. (Matthew 6:34 NIV)

Today's Prayer

Lord, help me to rely on you for the comfort I need when I am plagued by the unknowns of my life. Help me to take interest in my health, to have the capacity to learn, and to adhere to the education I am given. Give me courage and hope when I meet obstacles and when I have setbacks. Jesus, it is *you* whom I place my trust. Amen.

Chapter 30

Pain and Tingling
Is This Normal?

I notice that I have a pins and needles sensation in my feet. Sometimes, I'm not sure I'm standing, except for the fact that I know I am upright and on my feet. This can't be normal. I've also experienced a similar feeling in my fingertips during my treatment. It has been so painful that I have signed off treatment early. My fingers are cold and ache so deeply. I don't always have this, and it doesn't seem to be predictable. I have heard my fellow dialysis mates speak of similar experiences, so I guess this is all part of hemodialysis, right?

Week 30

There are some unavoidable discomforts associated with hemodialysis. There is pain associated with needle insertion. The needles are large bore, and the skin is tender, especially when first starting dialysis. Your skin will become less sensitive with time, but the pain doesn't disappear completely. All pain experienced needs to be addressed with your provider. Pain and coldness in your access extremity can be a warning sign for a narrowing or stenosis of your vein or artery, and this is correctable. Thus, it is important not to ignore. Other pains may be related to long-term dialysis or other health conditions, but you should never assume this! Please address all pain with your team. It doesn't mean there will be resolution, but there should always be explanation.

Journaling Questions

1. *How do I know if the pain I am experiencing is normal?*
2. *What is causing my pain in my* _____?
3. *What can I do for this pain?*

Information

- Hemodialysis requires insertion of two needles (one in the artery and one in the vein) for each treatment.
- The needles are different sizes. Common practice involves starting with the smallest needle (seventeen gauge) and advancing to a larger one to achieve adequate blood flow and adequate dialysis. The largest needle size is a fourteen-gauge, but most patients can achieve adequacy with size fifteen. Note that the smaller the size, the larger the needle.
- Other than the initial needle insertion pain and an occasional needle repositioning during treatment, all other pain experienced should be explored further.
- Pain in the access extremity, especially if associated with swelling, needs to be addressed immediately. This is often a result of an infiltration.
- An infiltration occurs when the needle dislodges from the vein/artery due to movement of the limb or lines or due to an inaccurate insertion at the start of treatment.
- Infiltrations are painful but do not cause long-term residual effects. They are most times treated with ice application and removal of the needle.
- If you are experiencing numbness or coldness to the access limb, it may mean there is a narrowing above the needle insertion site. This always requires a fistulogram to diagnose.
- A fistulogram is a diagnostic procedure performed at an interventional radiology center. Dye is injected, and an X-ray is taken to check for narrowing. If present, it will be ballooned open and resolved.

- Coldness and severe pain of the access extremity can also be due to "steal syndrome."
- Steal syndrome occurs when there is not enough blood flow to the extremity due to the AVF or AVG. This will require a surgical evaluation.
- Steal syndrome often can be managed by reducing blood flow rate, the wearing of a glove during treatment, or a surgical intervention.
- Tingling and numbness of lower extremities is called neuropathy. It is common in diabetic patients, as well as those on long-term hemodialysis.
- Maintaining good glucose control in diabetes is a preventative measure in developing diabetic neuropathy.
- Renal neuropathy can occur in long-term HD patients as well. Adhering to your HD prescription is the best preventative measure.
- Neuropathy pain can be treated with medication. Two agents frequently used are gabapentin or Neurotin. A medication called Lyrica may also be used.
- These medicines must be dosed lower for hemodialysis patients. If not, they can cause confusion, irritability, and mental stupor.

Words of Comfort

You're not the only ones plunged into these hard times. It's the same with Christians all over the world. So keep a firm grip on the faith. The suffering won't last forever. It won't be long before this generous God who has great plans for us in Christ—eternal and glorious plans they are!—will have you put together and on your feet for good. (1 Peter 5:9–10 MSG)

Gina Novak

Today's Prayer

Oh, gracious and good God, may your word comfort me when I am in agony. Take away this suffering and help all of us endure when the moments seem unbearable.

Chapter 31

Baby, It's Cold Outside

Days like today are particularly difficult. It's blustery and snowing with the temperatures in the single digits. Part of me wants to cover up my head and stay in bed. The flip side of this is that I know what might happen if I cannot get to my dialysis treatment. I'm not sure what scares me most, the bitter cold or the real possibility that dialysis is closed, and I have to tough it out today without receiving treatment?

Week 31

Dialysis employees are essential for the unit to function. Severe inclement weather poses problems for staff, as well as patients. First-shift patients are scheduled to begin treatments by 5:30 a.m. This requires staff to be in the building by 4:00 a.m. Often roads are not plowed and ready for travel at these early hours. All attempts are made to be open for business as usual, but there are backup plans in place in case of extreme circumstances. Each unit prepares their patients for these situations so that all can remain safe when such conditions arise.

Journaling Questions

1. What is the plan if my dialysis unit is closed?
2. What do I need to know to remain safe if I cannot get to my treatment?

Information

- Dialysis facilities under the direction of the medical director will initiate back up plans in the event of predicted severe weather.
- The plans may vary slightly from unit to unit, but the premise is the same, to safely dialyze the patients.
- Backup plans frequently address how to make sure all patients receive their regularly scheduled treatments. Shortening everyone's treatment to three-hour sessions often accommodates everyone when harsh weather is imminent.
- It is rare for a dialysis unit to close. In the event that this happens, patients are referred to their emergency packet distributed to them annually.
- The emergency packet reinforces what foods to avoid, fluid restriction, and what action to take should you be short of breath or feel poorly.
- All should have emergency supplies at home in the event of a weather crisis. This is particularly true for HD patients.
- You should always try to get dialysis within three days of your last treatment. The best way to get ready for an emergency is to plan *before* one happens. Collect the foods on the three-day emergency diet shopping list. Keep them in a bin so you have them on hand. The list allows for *six days of food and water*.
- The three-day emergency plan is available on the websites listed below.
- The following food items will be needed for the three-day emergency diet:
  - four small cans of evaporated milk or three containers of brick pack milk
  - one to two gallons of distilled or bottled water
  - powdered drink mix (lemonade, grape drink)
  - small cans or brick packs of cranberry juice
  - small cans of lemon-lime soda
  - small boxes of single-serving cereal (no raisin bran)

- ○ one box of sugar, sugar packets, or preferred sugar-free sweetener
- ○ canned pears, peaches, pineapple, mixed fruit, and applesauce in four-ounce single-serving containers
- ○ eight small cans or pouches of unsalted tuna, salmon, chicken, or turkey
- ○ one jar of peanut butter
- ○ one small jar of jelly
- ○ one small jar of honey
- ○ three small jars of mayonnaise (you will open a new jar each day) or eight to twelve single-serving foil-wrapped packets
- ○ two loaves of bread (consider storing a loaf in the freezer and replace every three months until needed for emergency)
- ○ one box of vanilla wafers, graham crackers, animal crackers, or unsalted crackers
- ○ four bags of hard candy (jelly beans, mints, sourballs, lollipops)
- ○ one package of marshmallows

https://www.davita.com/education/ckd-life/emergency-preparedness-for-people-with-kidney-disease
https://www.esrdnetwork.org/sites/default/files/content/uploads/3-Day-Emergency-Diet-English.pdf

- Other personal emergencies do arise from time to time. It is in your best interest to know your facilities policy for rescheduling your treatment.
- Most dialysis units will work with you to accommodate your needs in order to prevent an ER visit whenever possible.
- The onus is on the patient to take initiative in rescheduling as there are limited slots for patients to receive treatments.

Words of Comfort

> Have mercy on me, my God, have mercy
> on me, for in you I take refuge. I will take refuge
> in the shadow of your wings until the disaster
> has passed. I cry out to God Most High, to God,
> who vindicates me. (Psalm 57:1–2 NIV)

Today's Prayer

I lift my anxious thoughts and all my fears. I trust you to carry me through turbulent times, through crises, through all storms that enter my life. For it is in your name, Jesus, that I pray. Amen.

Chapter 32

Understanding the Hierarchy
of Kidney Regulations

I have been receiving in-center hemodialysis for several years. I have been satisfied with my care. I have learned a great deal from the staff and feel like I have a good understanding of my disease and the treatments available to me. Some days, as any business, things run smoothly and flawlessly. Other days, there are bumps in the road, and things get over-looked. It is interesting to me that every so often, the staff are scrutinized, and everyone seems to be dotting their i's and crossing their t's, as they say. I hear words like "kidney commission, and the state is here." What exactly does this mean, and should I be worried?"

Week 32

If you have experienced a visit from the state at your dialysis center, it can be of concern to you. You have become familiar with the staff, and it is natural to feel protective of the ones who care for you. It is important to know some of the language and checks and balances surrounding the care you are receiving. Your social worker or facility administrator is an excellent resource for additional information.

Journaling Questions

1. *What is the National Kidney Foundation (NKF)?*
2. *What service does the NKF provide to me?*
3. *Are there other resources that I should be aware of?*

Information

- Today, the NKF participates in research that is helping advance knowledge about chronic kidney disease, treatment, and patient outcomes.
- The NKF continues to grow and conduct stronger and more effective programs throughout the United States and around the world, leading the fight against kidney disease.
- The goal of the National Kidney Foundation is to reach those at risk before kidney disease occurs and impact those in earliest stages so that progression to later-stage disease is no longer inevitable. Go to www.kidney.org for more information.
- *The Centers for Medicare and Medicaid* (CMS) regulate how dialysis centers provide care to make sure that safety and quality standards are met. If you have questions or concerns about the care you receive at your dialysis center, it is important to know your rights and your responsibilities as a dialysis patient. Go to https://www.cms.gov/.../GuidanceforLawsAndRegulations/Dialysis *for more information.*
- Additionally, state programs exist to aid in reduction of the personal financial hardships associated with end-stage renal disease. An example is the Kidney Disease Program in the state of Maryland (KDP) designed so that Maryland may provide help and support for its citizens whose needs are partially or wholly unmet by present federal or private support, or both, for end stage renal disease. More information is available at https://mmcp.health.maryland.gov/familyplanning/Pages/kidneydisease.aspx.
- The Dialysis Patient Satisfaction Survey (DPSS) is to assess renal patients' satisfaction with the health care they are receiving, including satisfaction with their kidney doctor, the nurses they see at the dialysis clinic, other staff at the dialysis clinic and at their primary kidney doctor's office, the physical environment at the clinic, and their health

plan. The questionnaire is designed for all dialysis patients, including patients who are receiving hemodialysis and those receiving peritoneal dialysis. The questionnaire is flexible enough to be used across the country and by both public and privately insured patients.

- The leading dialysis companies in the United States are Fresenius Kidney care www.fresenius.com, DaVita at www.davita.com, and US Renal Care at www.usrenal.com.
- Each of these websites provide a plethora of information for both providers and patients and are excellent resources for all.

Words of Comfort

And now, friends, we ask you to honor those leaders who work so hard for you, who have been given the responsibility of urging and guiding you along in your obedience. Overwhelm them with appreciation and love! (1 Thessalonians 5:12–13 MSG)

Today's Prayer

Lord, it is good that you provide for me in all ways. Thank you for all who care for us during our treatments. Thank you for the checks and balances that protect us patients and guide those caring for us. Let my appreciation and love be known to those caring for me, especially when my lips do not say that which my heart feels. Amen.

Chapter 33

Water, Water, Everywhere

Today, as I entered in the building for my regular dialysis treatment, I could tell immediately something was wrong. The waiting room was crowded, and there was much more talking then on an ordinary day. As my anxiety heightened, I quickly learned that "the water was down, and no one could be dialyzed." I didn't know exactly what this meant to me, so I sat quietly to myself and listened to the other patients for further clarification. There was a variety of grumblings. Some said, "This happens way too much." Others complained that they had a lot of fluid on from the weekend, and they wanted their full treatments. Still others sat patiently, saying nothing, and some left without speaking of their plan. I wasn't certain what I should do when one of the staff came and announced that the problem was fixed, and treatments would be starting in the next thirty minutes. He encouraged everyone to stay and wait, assuring everyone that they would get dialyzed.

Week 33

There are a lot of working parts to a dialysis unit, and unfortunately all of them may impact *your* treatment and *your* time. Some of the factors affecting your "put-on" time can be staffing, patient emergencies, mechanical failures, and now this, a water issue. It makes sense that these unforeseen situations not only frustrate you but possibly scare you. Hopefully, the information below will bring understanding to some of the jargon associated with the workings of the dialysis unit and alleviate any unnecessary anxiety.

Journaling Questions

1. *What information do I want to know regarding my dialysis?*
2. *What dangers should I be aware of regarding dialysis?*

Information

- The solution used to clean or dialyze your blood is reliant on the water supply. In most cases, this is municipal water.
- The water used for drinking, bathing, and washing is purified through a water treatment plant.
- Water treatment plants use several methods to make your water suitable for use. These methods, include first, sifting the water through a screen that removes large particles. Next, chemicals are added to remove additional smaller particles, which were not captured through the screening. Then the water is filtered through sand, which removes the chemicals. Finally, chlorine is added to remove pollutants and bacteria that still may remain in the water. Throughout each step, samples are taken to assure effectiveness.
- Additional water purification steps must be taken to make it safe and suitable for exposure to blood during dialysis.
- Dialysis water systems use multistep processes to purify the water. This includes increasing the temperature, increasing pressure for the water to flow through carbon tanks, which removes chlorine/chloramine. Next is a process called reverse osmosis, which removes all dissolved material. Finally, a deionizer, which removes any minimal particles that remain. This complex system assures that the patient receives ultrapure water for dialysis.
- There are a multitude of checks and balances throughout your treatment to assure that there has been no breakdown in the filtration system.
- Some of the alarms that you may hear during your treatments is to remind the staff to perform these checks and balances.

- Chlorine testing is done every four hours. Chlorine prevents bacterial growth. Too much chlorine can cause damage to your red cells called hemolytic anemia. If the staff fail to respond to the chlorine check, a system is in place that notifies the facility administrator, as well as the regional director. This process is taken very seriously.
- Water samples are also checked by the biomedical technician. These samples are checked for bacteria levels, aluminum, lead, fluorine, and other elements. There are government mandates on what are acceptable levels for each. These reports must be seen and signed off by the medical director each month.
- Excessive aluminum levels over time can cause encephalopathy syndrome and hemolytic anemia. Most dialysis centers check yearly aluminum levels on all patients.
- In the event that there is a break in any of the filtration steps, dialysis may be delayed, paused, or terminated. Be assured this is for *your safety*, and although inconvenient, it is very necessary for your well-being.
- It is likely that at least 10 percent of the global population suffers from CKD. Sadly, most of the patients who have access to dialysis treatment are those who live in developed countries. Those who live in developing countries do not always have access to dialysis due to insufficient water supply.
- Water overflow from the drain behind your dialysis machine is not uncommon. The drains can become clogged, and without warning, they can overflow. While the water overflow is of no danger to you or your treatment, it is an indication that the wall box/drain needs cleaned. It also is an inconvenience and requires the staff to mop up the water and schedule for the drain to be cleaned as soon as possible.
- Dialysis wall boxes are located behind each hemodialysis station. They contain connections for the dialysis machine to receive acid and base concentrates and treated water and dispose of waste products. This area is susceptible to microorganisms and biofilm.

- The wall boxes and drains need to be cleaned and disinfected according to each facilities policy.
- Both boxes and drains are predisposed to biofilms that can cause clogs. Scheduling routine cleaning prevents this from happening. There are a variety of cleaning products available for use.

Words of Comfort

> God is our refuge and strength, an ever-present help in trouble. Therefore we will not fear, though the earth give way and the mountains fall into the heart of the sea. (Psalm 46:1–2 NIV)

Today's Prayer

O Father, there are times when there is so much fear around me I don't know where to turn. So I turn to you. Help me to find peace in the protection your love guarantees. Thank you, Lord, for the competent and trustworthy caregivers you have surrounded me with. Thank you for giving knowledge to man so that water created by your hands can be perfect for my needs. Amen!

Chapter 34

The Worst Is Yet to Come, Isn't It?

I see my neighbor suffering in great pain. I'm not exactly sure what is wrong with him, but I see him deteriorating. He once came in to treatment greeting everyone along the way. I remember thinking to myself, "How can he be so happy coming to dialysis?" Now he struggles just to show up. I see the staff spending more time and energy with him. Is this what it looks like when we near the end? Is this the destiny for each of us?

Week 34

You have been on dialysis for nearly nine months. You have seen and experienced some things. One of the blessings and curses to the ambulatory dialysis clinic is that there is not much privacy. This is a blessing in that we become our own support group. Although it is true that for the most part, we just share cordiality and general well wishes, we are doing life together three times a week. It is noticed when you are absent. It's like the old TV show, *Cheers*, "Everybody knows your name." It is a wonderful feeling to be known. Likewise, with this comradery, we share each other's suffering. We are not blind to one another's bad days, deteriorations, and even death. It is a bitter and brutal reality check to the devastation and untimely death associated with CKD.

Journaling Questions

1. How am I supposed to keep up the faith and perseverance when death is so close to all of us?

2. *What am I supposed to do when I see a buddy suffering, failing, and deteriorating?*

Information

- Kidney failure life expectancy, like anything, depends on many variables, some of which you can control and others that you cannot control. Age, gender, genes, race, diet, lifestyle choices, what caused your condition (etiology), the type of treatment you choose, how compliant you are with your treatment prescription, all have an impact on the outcome of your life.

- The life expectancy of a kidney failure patient with an eGFR of ten milliliters per minute or less ranges from one to twelve months without treatment of any kind (e.g. dialysis, transplant, medications).

- Although the average life expectancy of someone receiving kidney dialysis is estimated as 4.25 years, many individuals live beyond this estimation.

- Maintaining a high-protein diet, keeping a balance of calcium and phosphorus levels, and avoiding hyperkalemia all will increase survival rates.

- Daily exercise or movement thirty minutes daily will reduce cardiovascular disease and improve overall well-being.

- Achieving optimal dialysis by staying for your prescribed treatment plan is critical to survival.

- Emphasis should be placed on enhancing the quality of one's life, not concentrating on statistics. You are in control of making healthy choices. This requires planning; it will not happen by coincidence. Choose to live well with CKD.

- Joy comes from remembering your blessings daily. Journaling about what you are thankful for is one way to keep you in the present, acknowledging how blessed you are despite kidney disease.

- There is a quote, "It is better to have loved and lost than never loved." I think this is true when it comes to investing in those around you. You are not in this battle alone; all those around you fight the same battle. Who could be better to offer and receive encouragement than those sharing similar footsteps?

- Offering support to one another during a hard day can look many ways. Perhaps lifting them in a silent prayer, perhaps a knowing smile, or perhaps a phone call, note, or small token of love. Even a hand on one's shoulder as you are passing by can bring comfort of unknown proportions.
- Spending alone time, quiet time pondering your own thoughts and beliefs about death is time well spent. This is valuable for *everyone*, not just those with CKD.
- If you find yourself in need of information regarding death, life after death or any unanswered questions, ask to see your social worker for resources. Also, this is an area that you can delve into with anyone whom you have a safe and trusting relationship.

Words of Comfort

Can any one of you by worrying add a single hour to your life? (Matthew 6:27 NIV)

Today's Prayer

Lord, lover of my soul, take away my worry and replace it with your peace which surpasses all understanding. Lord, I lift my neighbors to you. I lift my very own life to you. Comfort me when worries surface. When the reality of death feels close by, show up and let me feel your presence and give me rest in you. Amen.

Chapter 35

The Trials of Transportation

When I first started hemodialysis four years ago, my son would drop me off at the treatment center on his way to work, and then my granddaughter would pick me up and take me home before her evening shift at the hospital. I felt extremely fortunate that my family were willing and able to do this for me. Unfortunately, my perfect setup was short lived. I quickly learned that put-on and takeoff times are not an exact science. The unpredictable events within the dialysis unit translated to my family's lateness to work, which translated to their frustration, my guilt and seeking other resources. Our social worker helped me apply for mobility through the MVA. Although a great service, it is accompanied by a whole host of frustrations!

Week 35

Transportation can be a huge source of frustration for dialysis patients. It easily adds two to three additional hours to one's already long and exhausting dialysis day. Multiply this by three times per week indefinitely. This is just the tip of the iceberg of the associated time consumption. Most transportation services require a ninety-minute grace time on both pickup and return travel. Patients, however, do not receive this same grace period. So if you have a complication or there is any type of delay of service at HD, this can mean that transportation will *not* wait for you, and you must wait for another ride. This often takes several more hours. So a ten-minute difference in leaving the treatment area can result in four additional hours sitting in the waiting room, often hungry, and fatigued after a dialysis session. Inclement weather, traffic pattern changes, and accidents all can further delay transportation. Very few patients feel well enough to drive themselves. Very few have the resources to pay for Uber, taxis, or rely on family for this level of commitment. Transportation is a problem for dialysis patients!

Journaling Questions

1. *What are my responsibilities regarding transportation to and from the dialysis center?*
2. *What services are available to me?*

Information

- Patients are assigned a shift and start/stop time.
- These times require flexibility, much like appointments at any office.
- Emergencies and workflow disruptions can occur at *any* time.
- Your start/stop times may be changed for a variety of reasons. This may occur without asking your permission. These changes are determined by your facilities administration.
- If you need to change your shift or time, it is best to inform your administrative assistant and follow up within one week of your request if you have not had a response.
- Facilities may have different processes for how these requests are handled, so this is an excellent question to ask of your facility's staff.
- Mobility is a service that requires an application. The application requires you to complete a section, as well as your provider. Once completed, you must schedule an appointment with the MVA. You *must* take the original application with you to your appointment.
- Once you have your appointment with MVA, it can take several weeks for the service to be activated.

- For major changes in a facility's schedule, the staff will communicate with transportation and inform you of your responsibilities. Examples of this are road closures for city events, holiday schedule changes, etc.
- Your role is to be aware of how your transportation service works. Important information that you should be aware of is:
    - contact phone numbers (point person to make schedule requests)
    - time frame rules for notifications.
    - being at the designated pickup location at the designated time (not looking out the window for their arrival)

- Have backup plans for when the service is inoperable. It may be an emergency contact person who can pick you up or funds tucked in your wallet for a cab or Uber.
- Bring supplies that will offer you comfort when you are delayed (snacks, drinks, word search, phone/tablet, etc.).
- Know the phone number for your social worker and establish a personal relationship with them. They are well versed in resources, brainstorming problems, and contact numbers to report grievances.

Words of Comfort

Do not be dismayed, for I am your God. I will strengthen you and help you; I will uphold you with my righteous right hand. (Isaiah 41:10 NIV)

Today's Prayer

Lord, day after day, my patience is tested regarding transportation. My thoughts and sometimes my words do not reflect your spirit. I am discouraged and feel at the end of my rope and so powerless. God, it is only by your will that I endure. Give me your strength when I am weak.

Chapter 36

The Underlying Disease Yet Lingers

I am surrounded by wonderful, knowledgeable providers, who know kidney disease! Like most of my fellow patients, I still must contend with my underlying disease, the culprit of my CKD. For me, the cause of my CKD is diabetes. So even though my HD is going well and I am stable, my DM is still warranting careful monitoring. Poor decision making in my past has left me with vision issues and vascular problems in addition to my CKD.

Week 36

It is true that at the time of initiating hemodialysis, most of the emphasis is placed on this aspect of your health. Equally true is the fact that your other health issues require vigilant attention. For many, this is diabetes (DM). DM affects your retina, heart, and entire cardiovascular system. While learning the newness of hemodialysis, monitoring your glucose and all aspects of your diabetic care must continue. Sometimes it is difficult to know how to manage all of this at once. Additionally, there is overlap between providers; thus, it is most important that good communication is established between all of your providers. Your role is pivotal in this communication.

Journaling Questions

1. *How do I learn about the effect's hemodialysis may have on my other health conditions?*

2. *It is difficult to know which provider to call for which issue. Any suggestions?*
3. *What is my role in keeping all my providers informed about my dialysis treatments?*

Information

- Although you are seen by a nephrologist or PA/NP at your dialysis clinic at least monthly, it is extremely important that you maintain a primary care provider.

- Nephrology is a specialty, just like primary care. And although your nephrologist is seeing you frequently, their role is to focus on your health needs as they relate to your dialysis.

- Primary care will maintain responsibility for health maintenance, immunizations, and coordinating all your medical issues.

- There are areas of overlap, particularly regarding blood pressure management, anemia, and bone health. This is one area where your role is to keep each specialty informed of changes.

- HD centers will give you copies of your monthly "rounding report" to share with your other providers. This report shows lab results, current medications, and vital signs.

- You can also share the names/numbers of your providers with one another so that more direct communication can occur.

- Systems such as *my chart* is a great tool to help keep all your providers connected.

- Because DM is the leading cause of CKD, other services are offered at your dialysis center that can help you manage your DM. These services include monthly foot checks and quarterly hemoglobin A1Cs.

- Other causes of CKD such as systemic lupus erythemotosus (SLE) or lupus (a *chronic inflammatory disease*) warrant close monitoring by your rheumatologist in conjunction with your nephrologist.

- Lupus flares can make hemodialysis treatments more difficult due to the muscle and joint aches. Sitting for long periods can aggravate your pain and lead to shortening treatments. This increases the likelihood of uremia and other complications. Managing both chronic illnesses is a balancing act that requires you and your providers to communicate regularly.
- Medications used to treat your lupus can impact your residual kidney function. Nonsteroidal anti-inflammatories (NSAIDs), ibuprofen (Motrin), naproxen (Naprosyn), indomethacin (Indocin), nabumetone (Relafen), and celecoxib (Celebrex) reduce inflammation and are especially helpful for joint pain and stiffness, but they can reduce the blood flow to your kidneys and reduce the amount of urine you still produce. As urine output amounts reduce, more fluid intake restriction will become necessary.
- NSAIDS also can irritate the stomach and lead to serious problems like bleeding ulcers. Dialysis patients are already susceptible to gastrointestinal issues, so caution is warranted. Taking NSAIDS with food or prescribed protective medications may be necessary.
- Corticosteroids, such as prednisone, is commonly prescribed for lupus. Your doctor will try to keep your steroid dosage at the lowest level possible to avoid side effects. Acne, weight gain, hair growth, fluid retention, and a redistribution of fat, leading to a swollen face and abdomen but thin arms and legs and fragile skin that bruises easily, are commonly noted.
- Long-term steroid use can increase your risk of infection. Infections are one of the leading causes of death in people with lupus. Lupus patients with a dialysis catheter are worrisome for this reason.
- Osteoporosis, where bones become fragile and more likely to break, is also a steroid side effect. CKD also is associated with bone disease. Treatment of osteoporosis in CKD/lupus patients must be modified and addressed by both

specialties, weighing the pros and cons in the best interest of the individual patient.

- Immunosuppressive medications are used when steroids have been unable to bring lupus symptoms under control. Immunosuppressive drugs reduce your body's ability to fight off infections. Therefore, they increase the chances that you could get viral infections such as shingles (chicken pox or herpes zoster). Dialysis patients with catheters are at an extremely high risk for blood infections that can have fatal outcomes.

- Commonly used immunosuppressive medications are *cyclophosphamide* (*Cytoxan*), *methotrexate* (*Rheumatrex*), and *azathioprine* (*Imuran*).

- Polycystic kidney disease is hereditary and the fourth cause of kidney failure in Americans. There are two forms of the disease that are passed down from a parent. The two forms are autosomal dominant polycystic kidney disease (ADPKD) and autosomal recessive polycystic kidney disease (ARPKD).

- Polycystic kidneys have cysts that form in the kidneys. These cysts are filled with fluid and, depending on their size and how many there are, will change the size of the kidneys. In addition to changing the size of the kidney, the cysts can interfere with healthy kidney functions and, after time, lead to kidney failure. About half of the people diagnosed with polycystic kidney disease will experience end-stage renal disease (ESRD) and will need dialysis or a kidney transplant.

- Autosomal dominant makes up 90 percent of all cases of PKD. It is called *dominant* because to get the disease, a person must receive one copy of a dominant gene from a parent. Those with ADPKD will usually have no symptoms until they reach between thirty and forty years old.

- Between 60 and 70 percent of patients with ADPKD have high blood pressure. Fifty percent of people with ADPKD may find blood in their urine (hematuria). Urinary tract infections are more common in people with ADPKD and should be treated with antibiotics as soon as possible to keep the infection from spreading into the cysts around the kidneys. Antibiotics do not penetrate cysts, so these infections need to be treated right away.

- The liver (cysts) and the heart (mitral valve prolapse) can also be associated with PKD.
- Individuals with PKD should have routine follow-up with their PCP to monitor for the other associated health problems related to PKD.
- Human immunodeficiency virus associated nephropathy (HIVAN) refers to kidney disease developing in association with infection by human immunodeficiency virus, the virus that causes AIDS.
- If untreated, *HIVAN* causes a rapidly progressive renal function deterioration often resulting in *ESRD* within two to four months of diagnosis. Dialysis remains the mainstay of management, although kidney transplantation can be effective in those with controlled HIV disease.
- Pill burden becomes a source of frustration for those with HIVAN and CKD. Discuss this with your provider before it becomes problematic.
- Coadministration of antiretroviral medications and calcium-based phosphate binders (calcium acetate, phoslo) must be avoided.
- Significant interactions exist between antiretroviral medications and many blood pressure agents, particularly calcium channel blockers and beta-blockers. *Any* adjustment to your medications should be discussed with *all* of your providers. Utilizing a PharmD is of great benefit to you, as well as your providers.

Words of Comfort

I will instruct you and teach you in the way you should go; I will counsel you with my loving eye on you. (Psalm 32:8 NIV)

Today's Prayer

My deliverer, I rely on you for guiding all my doctors. I trust you to keep them mindful of my multiple conditions when prescribing and treating me. O God, I cannot know all there is to know about my diseases, but you are thy great Physician. You are the one who knows all there is to know about me. Grant me comfort in knowing you are orchestrating my care. Amen.

Chapter 37

Beware of Infection

When I first started dialysis, I was convinced that my kidney function would return. I know now this was the denial phase of my coping process. The staff, administrators, and my own doctor kept telling me how important it was for me to obtain a permanent access. I kept avoiding that decision until I got really sick. I remember it very clearly. I came to my usual treatment, got hooked up on the machine, and then it hit me. I got so cold my teeth were chattering like in the cartoons. But there was nothing funny about how I felt. I was given antibiotics and sent directly to the emergency room. I was admitted and told I had a life-threatening blood infection that had affected my heart.

Week 37

CKD is a chronic illness. Anyone with a chronic illness is automatically more susceptible to infection because of a weakened immune system. This means you can't fight off infections as easily as you did before having a chronic illness. It is reality of living with CKD. There are choices and actions you can take to reduce your risk of susceptibility. Following healthy life habits is extremely important in preventing infections. These include eating a balanced diet of fruits, vegetables, protein sources, and getting adequate rest. Eight hours of sleep is ideal and daily activities include walking, stretching, or bicycling.

Journaling Questions

1. What infections should I be aware of, and how can I avoid acquiring them?
2. How will I know if I have an infection, and what I should do?

Information

- A blood infection (bacteremia) is one of the more serious and potentially life-threatening infections that dialysis patients are at risk for acquiring.
- The biggest risk factor for bacteremia is using a catheter as your access.
- At times, a person's decline and failure of kidney function is abrupt, and it is not uncommon in this scenario that a catheter is your only option for hemodialysis access.
- Even when this is true, pursuing a permanent access as soon as possible is in your own best interest.
- KDIGO guidelines and CMS regulations recommend obtaining a permanent access within three months of starting hemodialysis.
- Signs and symptoms of bacteremia are usually hard to ignore. They can include fever, rigors, or shaking chills, low blood pressure, a change in mental status, nausea, and vomiting. It is important to notify the staff immediately if you experience any of these symptoms.
- Your clinical staff are experts in assessing for and detecting bacteremia symptoms. If they suspect it, they will obtain blood cultures and contact your physician for direction in administering antibiotics and/or sending you to the ER for a further evaluation.
- Bacteremia usually requires lengthy administration of intravenous antibiotics usually four to six weeks. Most times, it does require hospitalization but not always.
- When the infection affects other organs, it absolutely requires hospitalization.

- Endocarditis is an infection of the heart valves. This is very dangerous and may even require replacement of your heart valve.
- A common secondary infection that can occur after prolonged antibiotic therapy is Clostridioides difficile or C. diff.
- C. diff is a bacterium that causes diarrhea and colitis (an inflammation of the colon).
- Other risk factors to acquiring C. diff is being age sixty-five or older, a recent hospitalization, a weakened immune system, and a previous infection with C. diff.
- Treatment for C. diff is prolonged oral antibiotics. It is a treatable and curable infection but often depletes protein stores and causes deconditioning overall.
- CKD patients can also be at risk for cellulitis, especially if diabetic.
- Cellulitis is a potentially serious bacterial skin infection. The affected skin appears swollen and red and is typically painful and warm to the touch. Cellulitis usually affects the skin on the lower legs, but it can occur in the face, arms, and other areas.
- Cellulitis occurs when there is a break in your skin's integrity, allowing bacteria to enter.
- If cellulitis is not treated, the infection can spread to your lymph nodes and bloodstream and rapidly progress to bacteremia.
- Also, it is important to keep up with the recommended immunizations. Common illnesses like influenza, pneumonia, and shingles can have a devastating impact on individuals with CKD.
- Most dialysis centers offer annual flu shots and the recommended pneumonia vaccines.

Words of Comfort

Nevertheless, I will bring health and healing
to it; I will heal my people and will let them enjoy
abundant peace and security. (Jeremiah 33:6 NIV)

Today's Prayer

Holy One, who watches over me day and night, I leave all my cares and concerns in your devoted and loving hands. Let me not leap on to (the what if train) but to trust wholeheartedly in you in all circumstances. Help me to care for this body that you have created and let me glorify you with this precious gift of life. Amen.

Chapter 38

Me and My Access

From my very first consult with a kidney doctor, there has been discussion about obtaining a "permanent access." I had a surgical placement of my arteriovenous fistula (AVF) months before I actually needed to start hemodialysis. My understanding is that this is the ideal situation. It avoids the need for a temporary catheter and all the potential complications. Unfortunately, even being proactive and anticipating my need for dialysis did not result in an easy road regarding my access. I had to have multiple procedures, and, yes, even a catheter placement before my AVF was fully functional.

Week 38

As your kidney function declines, you will be referred to a nephrologist. This may occur as early as stage 3 when some of the complications of CKD begin to occur. One of the many things that will be discussed is options for renal replacement therapy, and if hemodialysis is a likely possibility, then obtaining a permanent access will be part of the discussion.

The purpose for early access placement is to prevent the need for a catheter placement, as well as to be prepared for hemodialysis when the need occurs. A vascular surgical consult usually occurs simultaneously with a procedure known as a vein mapping. This is an ultrasound to determine the size, patency, and blood flow within the vascular system of your upper arms. The decision to place a native AVF or a synthetic arteriovenous graft is left to the discretion of the vascular surgeon, as well as your own individual preferences.

Journaling Questions

1. *What is the difference between an AVF and an AVG?*
2. *What if I have the surgery and then never need to start dialysis?*

Information

- An arteriovenous fistula (AVF) is the preferred access in the renal community.
- An AVF has less incidence of infection and thromboses than the synthetic arteriovenous graft (AVG).
- An AVF takes approximately eight to twelve weeks for full maturation and to be ready to use. This prolongs the use of a catheter if dialysis is needed sooner rather than later.
- An AVG can be utilized between two to four weeks.
- AVFs are reported to last longer with less interventions required compared to AVGs.
- A person's anatomy is often the determining factor between having an AVF or AVG placed. Small or weak vessels may prohibit an AVF from being placed or maturing properly.
- AVGs are more prone to infection and clotting. When an AVG becomes clotted, it will require an intervention called a *declot*. A person cannot be dialyzed until the AVG becomes declotted.
- AVGs can last for many years, but an AVFs last longer in general.
- Infection is a major concern in CKD. Many things place the CKD patient at a high risk for infection. Repeated needle sticks, a weakened immune system from chronic disease, poor hygiene, and comorbidities like diabetes are some of the things that place individuals at higher risk for an access infection.
- Daily hygiene practices at home along with thorough washing of your access at each HD session can help prevent infections.

- You are your best advocate for the health of your access. Make sure you look at it every day and report any scabs, open areas, or redness immediately to the HD staff.
- Common practice for a suspected infection is to obtain blood cultures (a blood test for infection) and/or to culture any drainage.
- If you exhibit any signs of generalized or systemic infection, your doctor should be notified, and broad-spectrum antibiotics will be prescribed until the culture results are available.
- In some instances, an infected AVG may need to be surgically removed, and a temporary catheter will be necessary to continue hemodialysis.
- In some instances, a clotted AVG or AVF cannot be corrected and another permanent access will need to be placed. A permanently clotted access is not removed due the risks of complications being higher than the benefits (mostly cosmetic) achieved.
- Likewise, a permanent access that is placed and never used due to transplant will rarely be removed. It does not cause harm to you, and again the risks of complications due to removal outweighs any benefits that may be received.

Words of Comfort

The Lord keeps watch over you as you come
and go, both now and forever. (Psalm 121:8 NIV)

Today's Prayer

God, I place my trust in you when it comes to my access. Protect me from the possible complications. Give me endurance when I do encounter hardships regarding my access. Help me to have the discipline to monitor my access for warning signs and give the staff keen observations that will protect my access for all my life. Amen.

Chapter 39

Binders, Phosphorus and More

For so long, I haven't been eating, yet I've gained weight and feel bloated. Now since I've started dialysis, my appetite is back. Isn't this a good thing? I met with the dietician and have been given a list of foods I must avoid, things like milk and peanut butter and bananas and many other of my favorite foods. I'm not really sure what to eat.

Week 39

The diet topic can be as daunting as lions, tigers, and bears. Oh my! Eating is such a challenging aspect of living with CKD. In the beginning, patients often suffer with loss of appetite and nausea due to elevated toxins called uremia. Once dialysis treatments begin (usually within the first three weeks), these symptoms subside, and your appetite reappears. Although this is great news, it also requires an entire new set of rules. Healthy eating with CKD is *not* easy!

Journaling Questions

1. *Are there foods that I can never eat again? What happens if I do?*
2. *How can I get proper nutrition and maintain my health if I avoid red meats, certain fruits, vegetables, and nuts?*
3. *What about if I want to go out to dinner with friends/family? Should I no longer expect this pleasure in my life?*

Information

- Phosphorus is a mineral found in our bodies and mostly contained in our bones.
- Phosphorus is absorbed through the food we eat.
- Healthy kidneys rid the body of excess amounts of phosphorus, but in CKD, the phosphorus accumulates. This condition is known as hyperphosphatemia.
- Elevated phosphorus levels can lead to weakened bones and easier fractures, calcifications in tissues, heart, arteries, joints, skin, and lungs.
- It may cause bone pain and itching when elevated.
- Preventing and managing hyperphosphatemia is done by
    o eating foods lower in phosphorus,
    o taking medications known as binders that act like sponges to soak up the extra phosphorus, and
    o taking the active form of vitamin D (available as a pill or administered during dialysis).

- Additional medication is sometimes required.
- Longer dialysis is sometimes required.
- A surgical procedure to remove the four parathyroid glands is sometimes required.
- Normal blood levels for phosphorus should be between 3.5 and 5.5. This is checked monthly.
- Moderation *not* deprivation is the answer to good health. Take your binders with every meal.
- The allowed amount of phosphorus is one thousand milligrams daily. The difficulty arises in that many food labels do not list the amount of phosphorus, so this is acquired information that through the help of your health care team, especially your dietician, you will learn!
- You should expect a great deal of emphasis and discussion about your phosphorus levels. It is measured monthly. Sometimes you will have a blood level outside the desired

parameters. This does not mean you will have complications. It is a measure to help guide you toward better food choices. It will take time to modify your diet to achieve the desired goals.

- An elevated phosphorus level does not *hurt*. There are serious health issues that can result from consistently elevated blood phosphorus levels. Therefore, keeping informed and working directly with your providers/dietician are crucial to gaining improved understanding and, therefore, outcomes (i.e. blood results within range).
- Eating out is a nutritional challenge from many perspectives. Beverages often have free refills, making fluid restriction an extra challenge. Portion sizes are often above the recommended serving size. Sodium or salt content is typically extremely high. And certain food selections may cause a *blip* in your potassium or phosphorus levels.
- Knowing which restaurants and which foods to avoid takes time and education. Allow yourself grace and ask questions of your dietician.
- In general, avoid appetizers (high salt content), do not order fried foods, and potatoes. Enjoying dining out is important and, with a few modifications, is a reasonable expectation for all CKD patients.
- Other types of food to limit due to poor renal friendly options, include Chinese, fast food, carryout, all-you-can-eat buffets, and smorgasbords.
- A balanced diet of fruits, vegetables, and protein sources will provide you with adequate nutrition. A monthly albumin (blood protein) level is obtained and followed closely.
- Most dialysis centers have an oral nutrition supplement program to assist patients in maintaining adequate albumin levels.

Words of Comfort

> Whoever comes to me will never go hungry,
> and whoever believes in me will never be thirsty.
> (John 6:48 NAS)

Today's Prayer

Lord, it is you who nourishes me from the inside out. By your spirit in me, I will never feel deprived but fulfilled in every way possible. Forgive me and strengthen me when I lose sight of that which is important. Amen.

Chapter 40

More or Less

One of the more difficult challenges that I've faced on dialysis is seemingly not all patients are treated equally. I've noticed that some of my fellow patients leave much earlier than I, even when we get on our machines nearly at the same time. I've asked my provider if I can shorten my treatments and was told no because of my size. I am not overweight for my height, but because of my height, I require more dialysis. This just doesn't seem fair. My time is just as important as my neighbors. Help me understand.

Week 40

The average dialysis treatment time is three and a half hours per treatment. Average time, meaning some will require more, and some will require less time. Factors such as body surface area, residual renal function, access type and function, as well as other health conditions help determine the amount of time prescribed by your provider.

It is hard to sit for five hours thrice weekly when others are staying just over three hours. Monthly laboratory values are obtained to determine the adequacy of your dialysis. Your dialysis team monitors this closely and discusses it with you on a monthly basis.

Journaling Questions

1. Are there any steps I can take to reduce the duration of my dialysis treatments?
2. What are the dangers to shortening my prescribed treatment time?

Information

- Each month, a sample of blood is obtained before and after dialysis to determine the adequacy of your dialysis treatment to remove uremic toxins from the blood.
- By measuring this small molecule known as urea, we can determine if your treatment is working for you.
- This blood test is referred to as Kt/V. K is a constant depending on the dialyzer itself. T is the treatment time. V is the volume of urea distribution in the body, generally determined by weight and total body water.
- The minimum Kt/V is 1.2. The Kidney Dialysis Initiative for Global Outcomes (KDIGO) has set this national standard.
- Dialysis centers may set the Kt/V goal higher at 1.4. This has not been proven to increase life expectancy or decreases mortality rates but, in general, indicates better cleaning of uremic toxins from your blood.
- If the Kt/V measurement is consistently below 1.2, areas for improvement to be considered are
    - longer treatment time,
    - larger dialyzer size if your weight is >100kg,
    - reliable access (for example a fistula is preferred over a catheter), and
    - higher blood flow rate or dialysate flow rate.

- A general rule of thumb is for smaller individuals to achieve a Kt/V of 1.4–1.6, and for larger individuals, a Kt/V of 1.2–1.4 is acceptable.
- If your *received* treatment time is shorter than your *prescribed* treatment time, you are receiving inadequate dialysis. *Longer time on dialysis is almost always better!*
- Any time you choose to shorten your treatment, you will be required to sign a statement indicating you understand this is against medical advice. This is not meant as a punitive measure but rather due diligence on the part of your

team to assure you understand the risks of a reduced treatment time.

- Residual renal function is a term to explain remaining kidney function in those with chronic kidney disease. It is not measurable. Individuals who have residual function may still urinate, may require less hormone and vitamin D replacement, and may be able to have a lower treatment time.
- Residual renal function is most notable in the "new to dialysis patient" or the patient who returns after a failed transplanted kidney.
- Maintaining residual renal function is best achieved by minimizing exposure to nephrotoxins such as
  o contrast media for diagnostic tests,
  o antibiotics,
  o nonsteroidal anti-inflammatories (NSAIDS), and
  o medication properly dose adjusted for impaired renal function.

- Individuals with severe congestive heart failure (CHF) or individuals experiencing profound cramping and low blood pressure during treatment may also require increased treatment times.

Words of Comfort

Be joyful in hope, patient in affliction, faithful in prayer. (Romans 12:12 NIV)

Today's Prayer

Father, hear my prayers for endurance and perseverance when my treatment time feels long and unbearable. Give me patience and understanding when I see others leave before me, and I long to follow. O Father, remind me of the many reasons that staying for my full treatment time is more important than the temptations that seize my heart and make me want to leave early. Amen.

Chapter 41

Am I a Disabled Person Now?

When I came to terms with my CKD and the requirements of hemodialysis three times a week, it was only part of appreciating my new reality. Being gainfully employed and a significant contributor to my family's survival meant that I worked full-time. As my CKD progressed over the years, I ignored the impact that my disease would have on my work abilities. Now it was here. I could no longer ignore that my livelihood was about to be impacted. I was afraid of what this would mean. Up until now, disability seemed like a service for those severely limited in their abilities. Was this my new reality?

Week 41

Working with the chronic condition of CKD is not impossible, but it does require flexibility on the part of your employer and perhaps certain work restrictions. Most of us want to have as few disruptions in our lifestyle as possible. CKD patients requiring in-center dialysis means you will need a work schedule that accommodates your treatments. There are three, sometimes four, shifts available when considering how to maintain your employment. Additionally, your employer may need to accept lifting restrictions if you have an arm or leg AVF/AVG. Usually lifting greater than twenty-five pounds is restricted. The other unpredictable factor is how you will feel in your job capacity once beginning HD. If you have some leniency by your employer, this is quite helpful initially.

Gina Novak

Journal Questions

1. *What must I do to apply for disability?*
2. *May I still work part-time if I receive disability benefits?*
3. *Who is the best resource for these questions?*

Information

- If you have CKD and require dialysis, you qualify for disability from SSA.
- If have had a kidney transplant less than one year ago, you qualify for disability from SSA.
- Older adults may have an even greater advantage since advancing age can be a limiting factor in an applicant's ability to adjust or transition to a new job.
- Maintaining a job with CKD is most easily achieved with sedentary job roles. Jobs that require excessive standing or strenuous activity would not be recommended.
- Applying for disability benefits from SSA is complex. Enlist the help of your HD social worker, your human resource department, and in some cases, legal counsel.
- Utilize the SSI disability advocates that are available to you. It will be helpful to know what your financial needs are prior to meeting with the SSA. They are in the best position to advise you on working while collecting SS benefits.
- Counseling may be helpful if you are considering termination of employment. This is a loss that often impacts individuals psychologically more than anticipated. Consult with your social worker for qualified counselors.
- Home modalities are a viable option for those concerned about leaving their places of employment. Both home hemodialysis and peritoneal dialysis give greater autonomy and flexibility for those wishing to work outside the home.
- There is greater emphasis on home modalities and transplant. The goal is 80 percent of individuals requiring hemodialysis would choose home modalities or be trans-

planted by 2025. This executive order was signed in July 2019 by President Trump and is called *Advancing American Kidney Health (AAKH)*.

Words of Comfort

They are foundational words, words to build a life on. Rain poured down, the river flooded, a tornado hit but nothing moved that house. It was fixed to the rock. (Matthew 7:24–25 MSG)

Today's Prayer

My God, I place my future in your hands. So many unknowns that keep my thoughts in constant turmoil. So much at stake! Lord, I stake my future in your capable hands. May my faith sustain the turmoil within me. I cling to you, my rock. Amen.

Chapter 42

I'm Back

There is no greater feeling than receiving the call that a kidney is waiting for you. Yes, there is some degree of fear of what lies ahead, but it is accompanied by this incredible sensation of hope! Could it be? Will I have my life back? With hope, everything is better. I wish hope for all of you reading this today.

There are many, many transplant success stories. Unfortunately, that is not my story. I received a deceased donor transplant kidney (DDTK). The surgery and postoperative process went well. I felt great, and my nephrologist took a picture of my urine output that first day. That probably sounds weird, but seeing her joy over my transplant made me feel wonderful. It almost seemed that the transplant was equally important to her. Who knew "pee" could make us so happy?

Six months after my transplant, I developed brown urine, and it became increasingly difficult to urinate. I soon learned that I had BK virus, and it was attacking my new kidney. Despite diligent care by my transplant team, my new kidney failed against this virus. I was devastated.

I had recalled nearly skipping out of the dialysis center when I got my call that a kidney was waiting. Now I returned like a dog slumped over with his tail between his legs. I was a ball of emotion. I was angry, disappointed, embarrassed, and feeling despondent.

Week 42

Whether you are this person described above or you have observed someone with this story, it simply adds to the sadness that can accompany CKD. Kidney transplantation is the *only cure* for CKD stage 5, but it is not always the end of the journey. Transplants do fail. This means a return to some form of renal replacement therapy, often in-center hemodialysis. It is a physically and emotionally challenging time for the individual. Often the staff will not know what you have just been through. If you return to your former center, others may ask you all kinds of questions, questions you are not prepared to answer or just don't want to. This is a time to extend grace to yourself. Be kind and patient with yourself.

Journaling Questions

1.   *What do I do now?*
2.   *What are my options?*
3.   *What resources are available to help me cope/start over/process all of this?*

Information

- A kidney transplant can improve one's quality of life and, for most, reduces the mortality risk when compared to those receiving dialysis.
- Postoperatively, patients will be on complex immunosuppressive regimens. This significantly increases their risk to infection, malignancy, and cardiovascular disease (CVD).
- Individualized treatment plans are developed for each patient consisting of frequent blood work and follow up by transplant nephrologists. Immunosuppressant agents are tapered slowly to avoid untoward side effects while preventing rejection.
- Routine blood work along with glucose levels, medication levels, urine protein, and GFR are monitored closely for signs of renal function.
- A renal biopsy may be performed if any signs of rejection are detected.

- Common medications include steroids such as prednisone, calcineurin inhibitors such as tacrolimus or cyclosporine, and antimetabolic agents such as mycophenolate or azathioprine. Other agents may also be prescribed.
- Infections are a major cause for failed kidney transplants. These are most common in the first several months after transplant.
- Types of infections can range from common upper respiratory infections and urinary tract infections to more complex infections.
- Transplant patients are monitored for cytomegalovirus (CMV), polyomavirus (BK virus), nocardia asteroides, listeria monocytogenes, aspergillus fumigatus, pneumocystis carinii pneumonia (PCP), hepatitis B and C viruses, herpes simplex virus, varicella-zoster virus, Epstein-Barr virus, and Mycobacterium tuberculosis.
- This monitoring includes routine lab testing to medicating prophylactically.
- Transplant patients are also monitored closely for cardiovascular diseases, lipid disorders, weight gain, and diabetes.
- In the event of a failed transplant, it does not mean the end of your chances, although it does mean returning to some form of dialysis for a period.
- Typically, your nephrologist at dialysis will resume your care after a failed transplant and assume medication management, but this may differ between facilities.
- Your eligibility for transplant relisting will be determined by the cause of your failed transplant.
- It is completely expected to have a host of emotions associated with the entire process. Be gentle with yourself. Counseling is available should you need additional support during the transition.

Gina Novak

Words of Comfort

> So also, you have sorrow now, but I will see
> you again, and your hearts will rejoice, and no one
> will take your joy from you. (John 16:22 ESV)

Today's Prayer

Jesus, my heart breaks. I am devastated that I have returned full circle and am starting all over. Give me courage and comfort, Lord, especially when I walk through the doors of hemodialysis again. Carry my burden, which feels too heavy for me. Heal my body of all that it has been through and give me joy again. This I pray. Amen.

Chapter 43

Blood, Bones, and Binders

Every week, I hear about my binders! Am I taking them with every meal? Do I need more? Am I snacking? What am I snacking on? And am I taking binders with my snacks? Is that snack you are having now low in phosphorus? Do you have your binders with you? Okay, you get the idea. I am driving home the point that these types of conversations get monotonous. I appreciate the importance of the blood results, and that taking my medications is imperative to making my blood work look good, but I am so tired of this conversation!

Week 43

As this first year of dialysis is fast approaching, you may find that you have stabilized. Your fluid status is under control, you feel better, your permanent access is working well, and your catheter has been removed. It's been a life-altering year with a great deal of change. It's natural to want to just coast for a while, to be still and rest. Unfortunately, having CKD requires on going *tweaking* and modifications of your treatment plan to maintain good health. These adjustments may occur every month depending on your blood work results.

Journaling Questions

1. *What can I do to keep my blood work in a healthy range?*
2. *The questions I have for my dietician are:*

Information

- The ideal phosphorus range for dialysis patients is between 3.0 and 5.5. Keeping your phosphorus in this range protects your heart, blood vessels, organs, skin, and bones from becoming calcified.
- When phosphorus levels increase in your blood, calcium levels decrease. This causes the parathyroid glands to produce a hormone (parathyroid hormone) to correct this imbalance.
- The higher the parathyroid hormone level becomes (iPTH), the more calcium is pulled from the bones in effort to correct the imbalance.
- When the iPTH level is elevated the condition is called secondary hyperparathyroidism or SHPT.
- SHPT is treated with a combination of medications: vitamin D, binders, and calcimimetics.
- When SHPT is not controlled with these medications, surgery to remove the parathyroid glands may be recommended.
- Untreated hyperphosphatemia or SHPT can lead to calcifications of your heart, blood vessels, organs, and skin. Leaving your bones brittle and weak.
- Vitamin D and calcimimetics can be given orally as a home medication or intravenously at the hemodialysis centers. The choice will be determined by your provider depending on your levels and how they are trending.
- Reading food labels and steering away from items which contain hexametaphosphate, sodium polyphosphate, dicalcium phosphate, tricalcium phosphate, and sodium phosphate will be especially helpful in maintaining a healthy phosphorus level.
- Phosphate binders are medications taken with meals that act like sponges in your digestive system to soak up excessive phosphorus so that your body does not absorb it.

- There are many options of binders. Your prescriber and dietician will choose the best alternative based on your individual labs.
- Options are sevelamer (Renvela), calcium acetate (phoslo, phoslyra), lanthum acetate (Fosrenol), Auryxia (ferric citrate), velphoro (sucroferric oxyhydroxide), and calcium carbonate (TUMS).
- All binders must be taken when you eat. They do not provide any benefit if taken hours before or hours after you consume food. They provide no benefit if taken on an empty stomach.
- Calcium based binders (phoslo/phoslyra/TUMS) may cause constipation.
- Renvela may cause GI disturbances such as loose stools or diarrhea.
- Common food items to avoid due to high phosphorus content are milk/milk-based foods, nuts, beans, chocolates, certain red meats, and dark sodas.
- Snacks can be a significant source of phosphorus in your diet. Some of the *worst* snack choices to *avoid* are cheese and peanut butter sandwich crackers, nuts and peanuts, snack cakes (Little Debbies), Snickers, Reeses, Mary Jane's, Cheez-Its, potato chips, puddings, ice cream, and chocolate cake.
- *Great* snack options are unsalted pretzels, air-popped popcorn, grapes, berries, skittles, apples, applesauce, shortbread cookies, lorna doones, butter cookies, or animal crackers.
- A dietician is available and an excellent resource for all dietary questions.

Words of Comfort

No discipline seems pleasant at the time, but painful. Later on, however, it produces a harvest of righteousness and peace for those who have been trained by it. (Hebrews 12:11 NIV)

Today's Prayer

Lord, take away this weariness about food and medicine. Give me the fruit of your spirit, self-control. Help me to not be tempted by snacks that will harm me. Give me discipline to hear this information and to adhere to a good diet. Amen.

Chapter 44

What Are My Numbers?

As with any chronic health condition, knowledge is power. I learned early on to avoid the mentality of being a victim of my disease. I take ownership in knowing how my labs are going. I ask questions. I stay active in my care. I like knowing what concerns my provider has and what our plan is. It gives me a sense of control because I know my disease, and it doesn't own me.

Week 44

In the beginning, dialysis can seem overwhelming. There is so much new information about kidney function, and you may be asking yourself, "How did I not know all of this?" The kidney is complex, as are all organs. The body was designed of many parts that depend on one another to work properly. When one system is not working perfectly, it can affect other body functions.

Common conditions that result from CKD are monitored and discussed monthly. It you have not already discovered, your provider will address this quickly, so it is important for you to know which questions to ask. Here are some common issues that are reviewed:

- Adequacy or how well your blood is being cleaned.
- Anemia. This is addressed with medications, iron replacement, vitamins, and blood transfusions.
- Bone disease. Calcium, phosphorus, and intact parathyroid hormone numbers are reviewed.

- Nutrition. Blood protein (albumin) and weight stability are reviewed.
- Fluid status. Interdialytic weight gains and fluid removal rates are reviewed.
- Immunizations. These include annual flu shots, hepatitis B vaccination, and pneumonia vaccines.
- Hospitalizations, missed or shortened treatments. Looking for increasing frequency and trends.
- Foot checks. Particularly important for diabetics or those with neuropathy. An untreated foot wound can lead to serious infection. Serious infection may be prevented with early treatment.
- Medication Reviews. So it's especially important to know or keep a list of your home medications. Sharing all changes with all your providers is key to avoiding over medication and dangerous interactions.
- Transplant status. Have you been referred? Do you have questions? Are there medical conditions that prohibit this option?
- Options for PD or home hemodialysis. Has this been discussed? Are you interested but need more information? Are there reasons that this is not a viable option for you?

Journaling Questions

1. *Is there an easy way to keep track of all this information?*
2. *Who do I ask if I do not understand something? Resources?*
3. *How does my PCP get this information?*

Information

- Each facility will follow a policy on monthly blood work that must or needs to be obtained. This is in part determined by your medical director, company policy, and CMS guidelines.
- Laboratory results provide objective data that help guide your care and optimize your dialysis treatments.

- Currently, dialysis facilities receive payment based on a performance score. It is called the end-stage renal disease quality incentive program (ESRD QIP). CMS assesses the performance score and applies a payment reduction to each facility that does not meet the minimum total performance score.
- Facilities aim to meet the minimum total performance score, not only to ensure optimal patient care but also because their financial survival depends on it.
- The ESRD QIP looks at indicators determined by CMS that change fiscal year to fiscal year.
- Your clinical provider (nephrologist/nurse practitioner/ physician assistant) reviews your blood work monthly to assure that your care is optimized first and foremost. Your provider will also consider the performance score guide-lines to align with the dialysis facilities mandates by CMS. Because these performance scores affect your HD prescription, these may be discussed if it impacts you directly.
- The system is quite complex and, at first glance, may seem nonsensical to base reimbursement on blood work results. The simple answer to this program is that hemodialysis is expensive. CKD is a permanent disability and, therefore, is mostly paid for by Medicare. Under the ESRD Prospective Payment System (PPS) for CY 2021, Medicare expects to pay $10.3 billion to approximately 7,400 ESRD facilities for the costs associated with furnishing renal dialysis services. These services include outpatient dialysis services, including drugs and biological products.
- Despite the financial *motivations*, your dialysis center and care providers really do want you to do as well as possible. A good objective measurement is your monthly laboratory values.
- A KTV above 1.2 indicates you are receiving adequate dialysis. The ESRD QIP score is set currently at 1.4
- A hemoglobin value (HGB) between ten and eleven is the standard goal. The ESRD QIP score looks at the percent-

age of patients in the entire center to determine if the goal is met. Anemia treatment may require erythrocyte stimulating agents, iron infusions, and occasionally, blood transfusions.

- Bone mineral metabolism parameters include three separate blood tests: calcium, phosphorus, and intact parathyroid hormone. All must be within range to meet the QIP criteria. Treatment to manage your bone disease includes adjustment of your dialysate bath, vitamin D supplementation (oral or intravenously) and calcimimetic medication. Binders play a large role in keeping your phosphorus in range.

- Fluid removal greater than thirteen milliliters per kilogram per minute is a newer QIP score that affects most HD patients. This, as all the scores, are guidelines. The idea behind removing fluid faster than these guidelines is that it can be dangerous to your cardiac health over time. Your clinician will use great objectivity and expertise in determining when it is appropriate to supersede this CMS recommendation. Sometimes extra fluid removal is crucial to your well-being.

- Immunizations are offered at each dialysis center. Hepatitis B vaccine is recommended along with pneumonia and influenza vaccines. The QIP score is based on a percentage of patients within compliance with obtaining the recommended vaccines.

- Hospitalizations and missed treatments are tracked closely. If you are missing/shortening treatments or are requiring frequent hospitalizations, the unit will determine if you are stable or unstable and make recommendations about your treatment prescription and/or offer problem-solving counseling.

- Foot checks are for those patients with diabetes. Monthly foot checks are required by the centers to assess for any issues. This is performed by the registered nurses, and any findings will be reported to the patient and the attending physician.

Words of Comfort

> You were taught, with regard to your former way of life, to put off your old self which is being corrupted by its deceitful desires; to be made new in the attitude of your minds; and to put on your new self, created to be like God in true righteousness and holiness. (Ephesians 4:22–24 NIV)

Today's Prayer

Father in heaven, help me to recognize when I am trying to control my disease, my lab numbers, and my future. I want so to be in control of my fate, realizing, of course, that my disease progress is unpredictable. Give me discernment and grace. Give me understanding into this whole world where I feel ill-equipped and ill-prepared. Give me your strength and your peace in every step. Amen.

Chapter 45

Hope Amidst the Never-Ending Hurdles

Life is not easy. In fact, Scripture promises that in this life, we will have problems. You would think living with CKD and hemodialysis three times a week as my only means of survival, well, that maybe would be enough? As a long-time survivor on hemodialysis, I have had my share of hurdles. I developed renal cell cancer after all these years. I withstood loss of part of my foot from diabetes complications, and now I am facing another health issue. Finding a source of hope among all the trials has not always been easy. I will not lie; there are days when I am just so tired of doing battle. My advice, if you want to survive well, you need to do the hard work of finding out where your hope comes from!

Week 45

Not unique to those living with CKD, the longer life you live, the more potential for additional health challenges. Much like an automobile or appliance, our warranty is limited. Not to sound glib, but growing older is not easy. A friend, an octogenarian at the time, told me that growing old is not for sissies. It takes courage and faith. Specifically, for those with CKD, as time marches on, you will notice some challenges that once did not exist. Although not a comprehensive list, your residual kidney function will lessen. This means watching your fluids more closely, perhaps requiring additional medications to manage your anemia and bone disease. Your blood pressure medications may need adjusted due to more noticeable side effects. You may need longer dialysis times, even though you feel like you can tolerate the sitting less and less. Dwelling on what is to come is of little benefit, but being prepared can take the element of surprise out of the equation.

Journaling Questions

1. *How can I address the rapidly occurring changes in my health?*
2. *Do I have a say on what I am willing to accept? How do I make my wishes known and nonnegotiable?*

Information

- Having a chronic illness like CKD poses limitations on your lifestyle in many ways. Many of the losses occur immediately such as your loss of freedom due to your need for dialysis.
- It can be difficult to verbalize the degree of loss you are experiencing. The HD unit does not foster a private setting to discuss the intimate details of your loss with your providers. But ignoring the loss is not a healthy approach either.
- HD units have licensed certified social workers who can help you acknowledge some of your losses and advise you on the next steps toward processing this enormous life change.
- Losses commonly experienced with CKD are energy, sleep, eating, sexual function, income, independence, self-esteem, and hope. It is a whole lot to process alone.
- Experts have reported that living with multiple and repetitive losses can morph into chronic sorrow or sadness.
- Because there is no cure for CKD outside of transplant, the person with CKD needs to set realistic goals for functioning as well as possible to live a quality life.

- The need for emotional support is not always acknowledged by your provider and seeking support services may not seem natural for you.
- Emotions that do not get addressed can lead to worsening health, depression, and anxiety.
- Journaling is one way to help facilitate and process your feelings to determine what is working and what is not working well for you. It is also a safe way to address your resentment, frustrations, and losses.
- Additionally, spouses, partners, and children are experiencing some degree of loss as well. Roles may have changed within relationships. Talking with your family about how they are coping with your illness is territory worth exploring.

Words of Comfort

> But I trust in your unfailing love; my heart rejoices in your salvation. I will sing the Lord's praise, for he has been good to me. (Psalm 13:5–6)

Today's Prayer

Hear me, Lord, when I cry out in despair. Hear my pleas for hope when nothing seems the same anymore and when I feel like I am the only one who is struggling with this disease. Help me reach out for help and not think that I can do this alone. Bring to me and my loved one's comfort. Place the right people in my path that can help me as I face so much loss. Amen.

Chapter 46

Skin Discoloring, Itches, Bumps, and Bruises

I was not prepared for the effect that CKD would have on my physical appearance. I have never considered myself vain, but no one likes to look unattractive. In all of my conversations, both before and after starting dialysis, no one told me about how my skin would become darker, or that I could be ravaged by sudden intense itching, or that I would develop bumps, bruises, and thin skin on my arm from the needles. I know now that it is just another part of life with CKD on hemodialysis. Warning! Be prepared and learn how to reduce or prevent some of these undesirable changes.

Week 46

It is true there are so many things to discuss regarding your health surrounding CKD that some things, even important physical changes, may get glossed over or completely omitted. I once had a patient ask me why there was not a book to prepare patients for everything. Excellent question, and in part, why this book has been written.

The skin, too, is affected by CKD. None of these changes are life-threatening or critical, but they are important and certainly warrant discussion. Although many of the changes are unpredictable and not completely preventable, there are some tips to try and reduce the severity of the changes.

Journaling Questions

1. *What causes the darkening of my skin? How can I prevent it, treat it, or deal with it?*
2. *My appearance is important to me. Is there anyone who specializes in treating these physical changes? I do not think I can accept them. There must be something I can do.*

Information

- Itching skin, known as pruritis, is a common issue for those with CKD. The most common reason for this symptom is a high phosphorus level. Phosphate binder compliance at meals and snacks, along with attending all treatments is key to maintaining your phosphorus level within an acceptable range.
- Pruritis can also result from allergies. On occasion, individuals have reactions to dialyzers. Rinsing the dialyzer prior to treatment often resolves the reaction, but if not, there are other dialyzers that can be ordered.
- Medications, such as Benadryl, may be suggested to help with the itching. Side effects such as sleepiness may limit this as a good choice for nighttime pruritis only.
- Topical creams have little systemic side effects and can be used on an as need be basis more frequently.
- Dry skin, known as xerosis, is also common with CKD. The theory is that kidney disease can change the sweat and oil glands resulting in dry skin. Dry skin for any reason usually leads to itching.
- There is not one sure treatment for xerosis, but many helpful suggestions such as avoid hot showers, using lotions, soaps, laundry detergent with fewer perfumed scents, and trying moisturizing soaps/body washes. Soaps and body washes containing oatmeal have been reported soothing to some.
- Avoiding lotions with high-alcohol content is best. Alcohol-based products can dry your skin more. Also, applying

lotions while your skin is still damp from showering will help it to absorb and soften your skin.

- Darkening of the skin, known as hyperpigmentation, is common to those with CKD as well. Urochromes are pigments that cannot be excreted. This can result in a darker appearance of the skin. Most patients are troubled by the change in their facial coloring. There are skin-lightening products and makeups that can be used. The results vary from patient to patient, so no one product is considered superior to others. Unfortunately, it is a trial and error situation.
- If you notice a white discoloring on your skin, this can be a sign of inadequate dialysis. The skin discoloring in this situation is known as uremic frost. This can be prevented by adhering to your full treatment times and not missing any treatments.
- Bruising can occur from the needle insertions/removals at such frequency.
- Hematomas or a large collection of blood under the skin can also occur. It may be tender and discolored for seven to ten days. It occurs from an improper needle insertion, a dislodged needle, or an infiltration.
- An infiltration occurs when a needle punctures your fistula or graft but then extends through it and blood leaks into the skin. This will cause you pain, and you need to alert the staff immediately.
- The needle will need to be pulled, and ice will be applied to the site. You will be instructed to apply ice and heat alternately once you return home. This experience, although disconcerting, does not result in long-term issues.
- Aneurysms can occur in fistulas, and pseudo aneurysms can occur in grafts. They occur due to weakening of the vessel wall from repeated needle insertions. The best prevention is the rotating of needle sites.
- Rotating needle sites are done by choosing a different site each time a needle is inserted. Some individuals follow a

specific pattern of rotation. The staff are trained to alternate needle sites as part of standard practice as well.

- Aneurysms can be problematic if the covering skin becomes thin or if they increase in width. If either of these issues occur, there is a high risk of spontaneous bleeding or rupture.
- The "unsightly appearance" of aneurysms can cause patients distress. They look like large bumps beneath the skin. They can be resected through ambulatory surgery for cosmetic reasons.

Words of Comfort

> For the Lord sees not as man sees: man looks at the outward appearance, but the Lord looks at the heart. (1 Samuel 16:7 ESV)

Today's Prayer

Jesus, help me to remember that I am beautiful in your eyes. Let me not be dismissive of how you see me and forgive me when I criticize my appearance. I am your creation. I have been made perfectly in your image. Relieve me of the discomforts of my skin and make me rejoice in you. Amen.

Chapter 47

My Chair
The Love-Hate Mystery

There are simple things that foster comfort. Maybe it comes from familiarity or our experience of them, but the attached emotion is real. I am quirky perhaps, but my dialysis chair falls into this category of comfort. It wreaks havoc on my emotion, attitude, and, yes, comfort when I find I will not be sitting in my normal chair. I get the rationales provided, the patient before me is still bleeding, and so that I can get my full treatment, I need to be moved. Or the machine at my station is broken, and there is already another machine ready to go at another station. The logistics I get; the emotion is hard to explain.

The funny thing is that sometimes, I loathe my chair! It's too hard. The air is blowing above my head. The patient beside me is too loud. Or a host of other reasons can stir up a strong disliking of my chair.

This mystery is real. It is like sitting in the same pew at church or parking in the same spot in the garage or sitting in my assigned seat when I was a kid in school.

Week 47

As the weeks of your first year of hemodialysis are marching on, there is a sense of familiarity. When the element of the unknown dissipates, so does some of the anxiety. Knowing what chair you will be sitting in, who your neighbors will be, how far you are from the scale, bathroom, nurses' station…all these things no longer have the element of surprise. So when you find yourself being directed back into the unknown, a feeling of discomfort is to be expected. Depending on other factors going on in your life, your thoughts, your world… this can be just enough to tip you over into full-blown panic or at least anxiousness.

Journaling Questions

1. *What can I do when I am faced with this dilemma? What is causing my anxiety?*
2. *How can I better prepare myself when I am placed in these situations?*

Information

- Mental health issues can surface in any chronic health issue. Patients diagnosed with CKD must deal with many difficult decisions in the face of significant morbidity and mortality.
- It is reported that one in five patients with CKD are diagnosed with depression.
- Depression in CKD can affect dialysis adherence, diet adherence, medication adherence, and overall life satisfaction.
- Similarly, anxiety in CKD can surface. Rates are reported varying in range from 12 to 50 percent.
- The repeated difficulties associated with dialysis and the loss of control are contributing factors to the anxiety experienced by dialysis patients.
- Anxiety symptoms can be exhibited in numerous ways. It often manifests in shortened and missed treatments, disruptive behavior, or worsening health.
- Recognizing that lack of control is a key factor in triggering one's anxiety, it is important for staff to explain all changes in routines as quickly and as effectively as possible.
- Because situations in the dialysis unit are unpredictable, it is not always possible to give patients a "heads up" on the changes.

- Unexpected seat changes, late starts, or unfamiliar staff all may produce an anxious response in the dialysis patient. It is important for both staff and patients to be aware of this possibility.
- Although explaining the rationale for these changes does not eliminate the feelings of anxiety, being given simple choices such as, "You can move to chair A or B, which do you prefer?" or "Your treatment will be late. You can wait, or we can reschedule you for tomorrow," can reestablish a feeling of control over an unexpected situation.
- As a patient, it is important to take time to figure out what your individual triggers for anxiety are and communicate these to the staff. Eliciting the help of your social worker may be beneficial in determining your individual triggers.
- Realizing that the presence of anxiety is unavoidable is helpful. Learning ways to deal with your anxiety makes the prison of anxiety optional.
- CMS guidelines require dialysis facilities to screen for depression/anxiety. This is usually done by the social worker when the patient begins dialysis and then every six months for the first year and then annually.
- Patients identified with significant depression or anxiety may be referred to their PCP or specialist for further management.

Words of Comfort

> Do not be terrified; do not be discouraged,
> for the Lord your God will be with you wherever
> you go. (Joshua 1:9 AMP)

Today's Prayer

My God, I get so alarmed when things don't go as I planned. My heart starts racing, I can't catch my breath, and I feel myself spinning out of control. I lash out at whoever is near. O Lord, take hold of my anxious thoughts, my physical reaction to my fears. Soothe away all my worries and replace them with the knowledge of how much I am worth to you. Fill me with your peace in these times. Grow me to trust you in all circumstances so that I expend no energy trying to control the impossible. Amen.

Chapter 48

Rest for the Weary

I would like to have a respite from HD, you know, take a few days off without having to give any thought to dialysis. Unrealistic, yes, but if you asked me how to make this life of dialysis better, that would be my wish. The professionals are very quick to empathize with my weariness of attending HD three times per week ad nauseam. The empathy is quickly followed up with a suggestion to consider home HD or peritoneal dialysis. Although these are great modalities for the right person, this is not exactly what I am trying to explain. I'm weary from it all. No, I'm not depressed; I am not done living. I am just spent from my circumstance of HD.

It is not good or bad. It is more of a "but-and-and" circumstance. I understand that I need hemodialysis to live; I want to live. And I want to stop dialysis because I am sick and tired of it. It's both. I am not looking for an answer; I don't believe there is one. There is nothing that anyone can do to change my dilemma. And it is my dilemma to traverse.

Week 48

As you are fast approaching your one-year anniversary on hemodialysis, you are more than entitled to owning your experience. It is not an easy to have your entire life's routine revolve around a schedule of dialysis. *And* though compliance to your treatment is essential to the best outcomes, the *but* to the hardships of 100 percent compliance is fully understandable. I would like to promise that you will not hear advice each time a treatment is missed or a reminder to what you could have done differently or better. The reality is that missed treatments will be addressed with concerned advice. The reality is that some days, the best you can do is own the weariness and nod in agreement.

Journaling Questions

1. *What is making me feel so tired?*
2. *If I plan to miss a HD session, what if anything can I do to minimize my risks?*
3. *What are the consequences to the dialysis unit if I miss treatments? Why is this seemingly so important to the staff?*

Information

- Weariness is defined as extreme fatigue, a tiredness, and the reluctance to experience any more of something, in this case, dialysis.
- It is important to rule out physical causes for weariness in the dialysis patient as it can be caused by a variety of things such as anemia and sleep apnea.
- Sleep apnea can disrupt sleep so often during the night that a restful sleep is impossible. This can lead to fatigue and weariness during the day.
- Your provider may recommend a sleep study if you are reporting symptoms of daytime sleepiness, fatigue, and an overall sense of weariness.
- Dialysis adequacy must also be confirmed if sleep apnea is diagnosed as high urea levels can be a cause.
- Sleep devices such as continuous positive airway pressure or CPAP machines may be prescribed. They help keep your airway open during sleep. Most patients report a more restful sleep and improved well-being and alertness during the day once treated for sleep apnea.
- Restless leg syndrome (RLS) is associated with sleep apnea. Patients with RLS also complain of fatigue and weariness. It too is seen in elevated urea levels, so receiving adequate dialysis is important in treating RLS.

- Symptoms of RLS includes a "fire ant" sensation that makes it impossible to keep your legs still. It has also been described as burning, pins, and needles or numbness.
- Anemia or low hemoglobin (HGB) can also cause fatigue. This is monitored very closely in the HD patient. Quality of life improvement thought to be due to less fatigue has been associated with keeping HGB levels between ten and eleven milligram per deciliter.
- In addition to physical causes of weariness, the mental and spiritual components should not be ignored.
- Mental exhaustion can happen to anyone experiencing long-term stressors. Whether described as weariness, fatigue or being emotionally drained, it is real and makes facing your responsibilities an overwhelming feat.
- Lack of motivation, social withdrawal, and calling out sick for dialysis are commonly seen.
- Unfortunately, most of the tips for managing weariness or mental exhaustions are not applicable to the dialysis patient. You can't just take a break, even though that is what you want to do! You can't just remove the stressor of dialysis. So what does that leave you with?
- Exercise, relaxation techniques, and emotional support are all options.
- Addressing your spiritual weariness may also be a key in improving your outlook. Spiritual fatigue can come from unanswered prayers, disappointments, and shattered dreams.
- Prayer, accountability partners, *fun*, and comfort scriptures can be a huge help when dialysis life becomes seemingly impossible.
- If *your* best decision is to skip a HD session, limiting your fluid gain to three kilograms, avoiding all sources of potassium, following a low-sodium diet, and remaining compliant with your medications will minimize but not eliminate the risk you are taking.
- It is advisable to schedule a makeup treatment in the setting of a missed treatment whenever possible.

- The clinical staff feel the impact of rescheduling challenges. It may require staff to work overtime to accommodate unscheduled treatments and downsizing of the staff are required when patients do not show for their treatments.
- Your facility does monitor missed treatments and financial initiatives can be associated with patient compliance.
- Poor patient outcomes are well documented related to missed treatments. These include death, hospitalizations, and laboratory abnormalities. Your clinical staff are responsible for giving you information and education regarding the impact missed treatments has on your health.

Words of Comfort

Yet those who wait for the Lord will gain new strength; they will mount up with wings like eagles; they will run and not get tired; they will walk and not become weary. (Isaiah 40:31 KJV)

Today's Prayer

O God, I beg you for renewed strength in my weary moments. Take away my fatigue, my weary spirit and help me to attend every treatment. Cast out the idea of missing treatments from my mind. Sustain me when I feel I cannot continue any longer. Give me the endurance to continue this impossible schedule when I just want to take a respite. Strengthen my character to do the best I can in all situations. Amen.

Chapter 49

Long Term Possibilities

Sometimes when I meet a new physician or a new person starting dialysis, they seem impressed by how long I have been on dialysis. I guess in some ways, this is complimentary to me. I have made it this long, fourteen years! According to statistics, the average life expectancy on dialysis is five years. I must be doing somethings right.

Unfortunately, just because I have survived beyond the expected, it does not mean I am living on easy street. Quite the opposite. Those with dialysis vintage, a cute term given to those of us being on dialysis for a really long time, are at high risk for a few things. I know, more bad news, right?

I have learned to accept my reality. I look at this way. The more days I have been given on God's green earth, the better. I realize that the older I get, the more health risks I am susceptible to, and this is true for all of us regardless of being on dialysis. But because of my CKD, I have a few unique health issues that I am prone to. Knowing this gives me no extra worry. Living each day, the best I can and to the fullest, appreciating each day as a gift from God, keeps me grounded and joyful.

Week 49

As a provider, one of the hardest balances is determining what and when to disclose information to my patients. Transparency is of utmost importance in developing a trusting working relationship between patient and provider. As I mentioned in the foreword, I am forever inspired by the grace and resilience I see in my CKD patients. My plan of care is individualized. Therefore, determining how much information a patient is ready for needs to be considered carefully. Too much information all at once can overwhelm and defeat hope in some individuals. Too little or holding back information can dissolve trust.

I approach the long-term sequelae of hemodialysis on an as need be basis. When an individual has dialysis vintage, I take this into great consideration when a person offers up a new concern. For example, if a patient develops a new joint pain and has not sustained trauma, I must consider amyloidosis as a possible cause. I explain this to the patient briefly as I am ordering tests to help with the diagnosis. I do not give an overwhelming amount of information until I am certain. I guess this approach has more to do with dealing with the worries of today rather than taking on borrowed and unnecessary worry for my patient.

Although this may not be every providers' approach, it is mine and has fared well in my years of experience. Of course, there are those rare individuals who need to know every possibility related to their condition. I find these individuals usually research on their own and come prepared with a list of questions for me. This is absolutely acceptable, and I am more than glad to answer their concerns to the best of my abilities with the information we have at the time.

Journaling Questions

1. *What future health concerns am I at risk for due to my CKD?*
2. *What screening measures or preventative steps are being taken to avoid these risks?*
3. *Are there any measures I should be taking to decrease my chances for dialysis longevity complications?*

Information

- It is important to remember that not everyone receiving dialysis for many years will acquire these problems associated with dialysis vintage.
- If knowing these risks heightens your anxiety, then skip for now and revisit should the need arise.

- Typically, the kidneys will shrink or atrophy with dialysis vintage. If a patient develops an elevated hemoglobin unrelated to medication, the provider is prompted to obtain a CT scan to evaluate for RCC.
- Routine CT scans for all patients receiving HD is not standard of care in screening for RCC.
- The risk of developing renal cell carcinoma (RCC) is estimated at thirty times greater *if* the cause for CKD is acquired polycystic kidney disease.
- Risk factors include smoking, obesity, HTN, occupational exposure to toxic compounds such as cadmium, asbestos, and petroleum byproducts. Genetics may also play a role in increasing risks.
- Adynamic bone disease is the most common form of bone disease found in dialysis patients. It is usually asymptomatic, but some will complain of bone pain. A higher risk of bone fracture is associated with adynamic bone disease.
- Clues to adynamic bone disease include vascular calcifications noted in imaging studies or hypercalcemia. This results in higher mortality.
- Persistent low iPTH levels is suggestive of adynamic bone disease.
- Risk factors for adynamic bone disease are calcium containing phosphate binders, high dialysate calcium, and the use of vitamin d analogues.
- Dialysis related amyloidosis (DRA) is a disabling disease caused by an accumulation of amyloid fibrils in the tissue and bone. These fibrils consisting of beta2 microglobulin (beta2-m) are normally cleared by the kidneys.
- Carpal tunnel syndrome, shoulder pain, neck pain, and pathological fractures from bone cysts are the most debilitating issues for patients.
- The use of high flux biocompatible membranes has helped clear the beta2-m. Dialysis duration and frequency also impact the clearance.

- It is standard practice to increase dialysis time for those suffering with DRA pain. Some recommendations for nocturnal or short daily HD may be better in clearing beta2 microglobulins.
- There is no specific treatment for DRA other than transplant. Over time, the deposits may resolve along with alleviation of the joint pain.
- Surgical intervention and pain management may both be necessary.

Words of Comfort

The Lord himself goes before you and will be with you; he will never leave you nor forsake you. Do not be afraid; do not be discouraged. (Deuteronomy 31:8 NIV)

Today's Prayer

God, only you know what lies ahead. Worrying about what could or might be is stealing my joy from today. Let me cast all my worries of tomorrow aside and set my focus on today. Lord, I trust you as my protector, my shield from all harm. I am faithful that you will never leave me nor forsake me in times of trouble. Amen.

Chapter 50

Putting It All Together

Dialysis simply put is just a way to rid our bodies of the things that are harmful to us. Too much of anything can cause us to get out of order. I know I am dumbing it down, but it is an easy way to remember why dialysis is so important to sustaining me. If I have too much fluid from the watermelon I ate, too much potassium from my french fries, too much phosphorus from my Coca-Cola Big Gulp, too much sodium from my second helping of Campbell's noodle soup, the list goes on and on. Too much for my damaged kidneys to handle! Dialysis is the only way to keep me in balance.

Secondly, in addition to cleaning my blood and removing the excess fluid, medications given during dialysis helps keep my bones from becoming too brittle, my red cells from becoming low, my iron stores from becoming depleted, and sometimes I may need additional medications to keep my body from excessive calcifications. Again, simplifying some complex processes, but I receive vitamin D analogues (synthetic active vitamin D), erythrocyte stimulating agents, iron replacement, and sometimes calcimimetics to keep my calcium in my bones and my parathyroid hormones at bay.

Dialysis is the only means to survive when your kidneys are functioning at 10 percent. There is in-center hemodialysis, home hemodialysis, or peritoneal dialysis.

Transplant is another viable option, but not everyone qualifies for transplant depending on other comorbidities or health conditions. Transplants can be received from a living related donor, a living non-related donor, or a deceased donor.

My chances for survival on hemodialysis are greatly impacted by the following:

- *attending my full dialysis treatments and not missing any*
- *receiving a permanent working access rather than a catheter*
- *maintaining my health by receiving preventative care from a primary care provider*
- *maintaining compliance with all my medications*
- *avoiding harmful substances like smoking, vaping, excessive alcohol, narcotics, or street drugs*
- *adhering to my kidney diet and fluid restriction*
- *receiving my recommended immunizations such as the influenza, pneumonia vaccines, and hepatitis vaccines*

Week 50

Transitioning to a life on dialysis is not an easy one. Hopefully in this last year, you have learned that you can lead a productive life that is of high quality. There are many resources available to you. You are surrounded by many highly qualified care providers who wish to support and guide you through this new territory. You have persevered and grown in this last year. Yes, your physical body has had to adjust, and your mental health has had to as well. Your spiritual growth has no doubt skyrocketed in ways you thought were impossible. You have been created with such amazing intricacy. Dialysis is simply one way to keep this well-designed instrument functioning to its fullest capacity. Be proud of yourself for all that you have endured. May you embrace your days to the fullest and let your countenance be a sign of worship to our God.

Journaling Questions

1. *The most important life lesson that I have learned from becoming a dialysis patient is.*
2. *If I could share one piece of information to a newly diagnosed dialysis patient, it would be...*

Information

- Give yourself grace and realize it takes most people six to eighteen months to adjust to major life changes.
- CKD and dialysis impacts every aspect of your life: daily routines, eating and diet, your work-life and finances, your vacations, travel, and holidays, family and friend gatherings and relationships, sex life and childbearing, exercise, physical health and appearance, and your spiritual life and outlook.
- Joining support groups and other social forums can be a means of encouragement to some.
- Utilizing all the available resources is encouraged. The internet provides easy access to great information sharing.
- Remember to seek reliable renal resources from dialysis organizations, Center for Disease Control (CDC), National Kidney Foundation (NKF), and your individual nephrologists.
- Reflect on your own growth by reviewing your journal entries and commend yourself for how much you have learned, endured, and survived!
- Celebrate your small and large accomplishments. Reward yourself appropriately when you have met your goals.
- Keep a list of your answered prayers to remind you of *how great God* is always in *all* ways!
- Refer often to your list of items that bring *joy* to you. Small visits to this list can make the difference in your day's outlook and get you through the rough spots.
- Pray often.
- Listen to uplifting music.
- Consider obtaining an "accountability partner" who will help you with the temptations that cause you to stumble.
- Have "go-to" phrases posted in your home, on your phone, or elsewhere that will give you encouragement frequently.
- Ask questions always.

- Develop a trusting rapport with your dialysis team. Tap into all the resources available. (Dietician and social worker are phenomenal resources!)
- Keep a record of all the many things that you *can do*! Satan will try and thwart your self-esteem by revealing inadequacies. *Do not* give him a foothold!
- Cast all your cares on your Lord. He is for you and *never* against you.

Words of Comfort

> Who, then, can separate us from love of Christ? Can trouble do it, or hardship or persecution or hunger, or poverty or danger or death? (Romans 8:35 NIV)

> For I am certain that nothing can separate us from his love: neither death nor life, neither angels nor other heavenly rulers or powers, neither the present nor the future, neither the world below— there is nothing in creation that will ever separate us from the love of God which is ours through Christ Jesus our Lord. (Romans 8:38 MSG)

Today's Prayer

Dear heavenly God, Ruler and Reigner over all creation, thank you for creating me just as I am. Thank you for being for me and not against me. Thank you for your divine order and planning in my life. Come, Lord, have your way in me. Keep my heart steadfast in hope and fill me with joy. Let me be a conduit of encouragement to those running the race with me. Let me fear no bad news but trust in you always. And, Lord, in those moments when my faith may falter and doubts set in, let me know that you, God, are surely in this place, and your way is perfect. Amen.

Chapter 51

Desperate for a Cure

*I am the fourth person in my family needing dialysis, third genera-
tion. Why has there not been any improvement in kidney disease? I have
vague memories of my grandmother needing dialysis at the end of her life.
I don't recall many details but know that it was hard on my own mom
as she watched her mom go through this. My recollection of my uncle's
journey (mom's brother) is clearer. He didn't always go to treatments,
was in and out of the hospital a lot, and died relatively young at age for-
ty-five. Now it's my turn. Great. I know diabetes is hereditary. I've done
what I've known to do, but here I am on dialysis, waiting desperately for
a transplant. Honestly, I just wish there was a cure. All of us sitting here
week after week would love to hear that modern medicine is closer to a
cure. Dialysis seems a bit barbaric when it seems that advances have been
made in other conditions.*

Week 51

Great observation! Even greater questions! You are right, the
advances in CKD have been minimal in the last several decades. The
major emphasis has been placed on prevention, educating the public, working with primary care providers to screen early and refer to
nephrology earlier. Currently there is much discussion on payment
plans. This has resulted in a bigger push for newly diagnosed patients
to consider home hemodialysis or peritoneal dialysis. Not only do
these options provide greater autonomy and normalcy to a person's
lifestyle, it is, in fact, a less expensive alternative.

Other advances have been in researching a "wearable artificial kidney," access placement via laser instead of surgery, and promoting engineering education in the field of medicine.

Journaling Questions

1. *How close are we to a cure for CKD?*
2. *How can I have a "quality life" while I'm waiting on a cure?*

Information

- *The bioartificial kidney* is about the size of a soda can. It will sit in the abdomen, close to the bladder, where it will perform the filtration function of the glomerulus. It will also dispose of waste and direct nutrients back into the bloodstream. While not yet confirmed, the device *is expected to deliver* GFR values of twenty to thirty milliliter per minute. The device is *designed to last* for years. If it fails, its filter or cells are reparable through minimally invasive surgery. Implantation will be like kidney transplant surgery. Once available to the public, it can be completed by a trained surgical implant team at any hospital.
- Although the kidney project and its technology are still at an early stage of development, the bioartificial kidney has recently been moving through porcine trials. It is possible that human trials could start soon, potentially leading to next steps and ultimately FDA approval. The time frame for this is dependent on several events, but if all goes well, approval could occur within the early part of the next decade.
- KidneyX is deploying several competitions. The first, *Redesign Dialysis*, focused on the development and commercialization of next-generation dialysis products. Redesign Dialysis offers a total prize of more than $2.6 million, includes two phases and seeks solutions that help replicate kidney functions, improve patient quality of life, improve kidney replacement therapy access, and strengthen

safety monitoring functions. For more information go to http://blogs.davita.com/medical-insights/2019/05/16/kidney-x-phase-1-winners-announced/

- Advances have been made on minimizing surgery for AVFs through interventional radiology procedures. This is called a percutaneous fistula creation. There are specially designed catheters that work by using thermal energy or radiofrequency energy to bridge the artery to the vein. The advantages reported are that it is a less invasive procedure as well as a reduced wait time for maturity and use. This procedure is new to the United States market but shows promise to advancing fistula formation in a less invasive and more cost-effective approach.

- Quality of life (QOL) is defined as the amount of enjoyment and satisfaction that a person gets from his/her daily routine. The social worker at the in-center HD units is required to assess your perception of your QOL annually. This helps identify issues such as depression, which can lead to poor health and poor decision making.

- Consider obtaining a job related to CKD. The Department of Rehabilitation is a good start https://*www2.ed.gov*/about/offices/list/osers/rsa/index.htm

- Consider doing volunteer work. There are needs regardless of your interests, animals, elderly, children, the National Kidney Foundation to name a few. Google searches are an excellent starting place.

- Consider enrolling in a class or taking up a new hobby. Most community colleges offer discounts or free classes to those with disabilities. Check out the websites at colleges near your home for available courses.

Words of Comfort

There's more to come: We continue to shout our praise even when we're hemmed in with troubles, because we know how troubles can develop passionate patience in us, and how that patience in turn forges the tempered steel of virtue, keeping us alert for whatever God will do next. In alert expectancy such as this, we're never left feeling shortchanged. Quite the contrary—we can't round up enough containers to hold everything God generously pours into our lives through the Holy Spirit! (Romans 5:3–5 MSG)

Today's Prayer

Father in heaven, let me make the most of every day, every moment, and every breath. Help me to see beyond my own needs and circumstances. Let me find ways to be a blessing to others despite my CKD. Provide me with opportunity to contribute, to instill hope to my neighbor, and to help those in need. Thank you for all the times you bring others into my life who encourage and lift me when I am desperate. Lord, I rely on your great healing in this disease. Bring cure in your timing. I beg that my children and my children's children will not carry this burden. Amen.

Chapter 52

Is This All There Is to My Life?

This is a reasonable question that we all ask once we've been handed the diagnosis of CKD stage 5 and learn that in order to live, we will need dialysis the rest of our life. To be honest, the first year after my diagnosis, I could barely think beyond one week at a time. I didn't give much thought to how all this changed my plans, dreams, and hopes. Eventually, the routine of living with dialysis does settle in, and then you will start thinking, "Is this all there is to my life now?"

The answer to this question depends on the attitude you decide to embrace. We can become the victim to this terrible illness, or we can do our best to contribute to our families, our friends, our neighborhoods, and our society. I've met some pretty resilient and faithful fellow patients, and their stories are amazing! Like the fellow who was faithful, he would receive a transplant, but in the meantime, he worked alongside the National Kidney Foundation, educating his community about kidney disease. One day, he even scaled an eighteen-story building as part of the NKF campaign. I love that picture of him, midair with the hugest smile of joy on his face. He did receive a transplant too. Another patient who continued to provide childcare for her grandkids, getting them ready for school, encouraging them with their activities, showing up at their basketball games, and doing life right beside them. One could wonder if this disease didn't give her even more determination to be present in their lives than if she were well.

Week 52

Dialysis is a treatment for a chronic illness. The good news, there is a treatment for CKD. End-Stage Renal Disease (ESRD) is the former name for CKD. End-stage…hmm, that does have a daunting sound and glum prediction for one's future. I have friends who have been on dialysis for twenty years! No, that isn't an average life expectancy, but it's possible, just like living a full and meaningful life is possible with CKD. Do not lose your hope. Dare to dream. Anything is possible!

Journaling Questions

1. *How do I plan to lead a life of significance despite this illness?*
2. *What might be the stumbling blocks and how can I overcome them?*

Information

- Some cruise lines cater specifically to those needing dialysis. For more information, go to www.dialysisatsea.com.
- If you have Medicare, 80 percent of dialysis costs will be covered throughout the United States. Some secondary insurances will pick up the additional 20 percent. Talk to your social worker about your benefits for travel.
- Air flight is not contraindicated for dialysis patients.
- Joining the National Kidney Foundation is free for dialysis patients. Go to www.NKF.org.
- Make a Wish Foundation is available to children with CKD. See www.makeawish.com.
- Employment is possible for HD patients. Some areas offer night HD so that you can sleep and be dialyzed in center at the same time.
- There may be monies/scholarships available for CKD patients to continue to pursue their education.

- Local opportunities exist to serve and educate others about CKD. Examples are participating in grand rounds at your local hospital, participating at NKF events, contributing to newsletters, or writing/sharing your own story on public forums.

Words of Comfort

> My grace is sufficient for you, for my power is made perfect in weakness. (2 Corinthians 12:9 NIV)

Today's Prayer

Lord, use me as an instrument to spread the word about kidney disease in any way you desire. I avail myself to you for greater purposes than myself. For I know that in my weakness, you are strong. Thank you for using me your humble servant to reach the many. Amen.

About the Author

Gina Novak's devotional writings are inspired by the thousands of patients and their families that she has cared for in her professional life. Her insights and reflections come from her experiences as an advanced practice nurse in the field of medicine. Her passion is to bring healing to those with chronic kidney disease and enhance the quality of their lives.

She continues to work full-time as a nurse practitioner in Maryland where she resides with her husband and two stepchildren. Her personal relationship with Christ is enhanced through journaling and being blessed by a strong support system, both inside and outside of her church. She credits her success and longevity in health care to deeply investing in others beyond the demands of their disease.

CPSIA information can be obtained
at www.ICGtesting.com
Printed in the USA
BVHW071239190821
614776BV00007B/122